Beat Excess Weight, Beat Unhealthy Lifestyle

A Comprehensive Step-by-step Guide to Lose Weight Effectively with Delicious 0 Point Recipes and Easy-to-Follow Workouts to Shed Pounds and Live a Vibrant Lifestyle (Illustrated Pictures Included).

CLARE A. DEEN

Copyright Page

TABLE OF CONTENTS

1. UNDERSTANDING WEIGHT LOSS

Weight loss, beyond aesthetics, encompasses a range of health benefits and considerations that extend far beyond mere physical appearance. While the pursuit of weight loss is often associated with aesthetic goals such as improving one's appearance or fitting into certain clothing sizes, its significance goes much deeper, impacting both physical and mental well-being. Here's a broader perspective on defining weight loss:

- **Health Improvement:** Weight loss can significantly improve various health markers and reduce the risk of chronic diseases such as type 2 diabetes, cardiovascular diseases, certain cancers, and metabolic syndrome. Excess weight is often associated with increased inflammation, insulin resistance, high blood pressure, and abnormal lipid profiles. Losing weight can mitigate these risks and improve overall health outcomes.

- **Enhanced Mobility and Functionality:** Carrying excess weight can strain joints and muscles, leading to reduced mobility and functionality. Weight loss can alleviate this strain, making movement easier and improving overall physical function. This can enhance quality of life and enable individuals to engage in activities they may have previously avoided due to physical limitations.

- **Improved Mental Health:** Excess weight can take a toll on mental well-being, contributing to issues such as low self-esteem, depression, and anxiety. Weight loss can lead to improved self-confidence, mood, and overall mental health. Physical activity associated with weight loss can also release endorphins, which are natural mood lifters.
- **Better Sleep Quality:** Obesity and excess weight are closely linked to sleep disorders such as sleep apnea and insomnia. Losing weight can improve sleep quality and reduce the severity of these disorders, leading to better overall rest and rejuvenation.
- **Increased Energy Levels:** Carrying excess weight can lead to feelings of fatigue and low energy levels due to increased strain on the body's systems. Weight loss can alleviate this burden, leading to increased energy levels and improved vitality for daily activities.
- **Longevity and Quality of Life:** Studies consistently show that maintaining a healthy weight is associated with increased longevity and improved overall quality of life. By reducing the risk of chronic diseases and enhancing physical and mental well-being, weight loss can contribute to a longer, healthier life.

- **Educational and Inspirational:** For many individuals, embarking on a weight loss journey involves learning about nutrition, exercise, and lifestyle habits. This educational process can empower individuals to make healthier choices and serve as an inspiration to others facing similar challenges.

In conclusion, while weight loss is often pursued for aesthetic reasons, its significance extends far beyond appearance. By improving health, mobility, mental well-being, sleep quality, energy levels, and overall quality of life, weight loss plays a crucial role in promoting holistic wellness and longevity.

THE SCIENCE OF FAT METABOLISM

Fat metabolism, also known as lipid metabolism, refers to the biochemical processes that involve the breakdown, synthesis, and utilization of fats (or lipids) in living organisms. It's a crucial aspect of energy balance and homeostasis in the body. Here's a simplified explanation of the science behind fat metabolism:

- **Digestion and Absorption:** The process begins in the digestive system where dietary fats are broken down into smaller molecules called fatty acids and glycerol. This breakdown primarily occurs in the small intestine with the help of enzymes such as lipase.
- **Transport:** Once broken down, fatty acids and glycerol are absorbed by the intestinal cells and packaged into structures called chylomicrons. These chylomicrons are released into the lymphatic system and eventually enter the bloodstream, where they transport lipids to various tissues throughout the body.
- **Storage:** Excess dietary fats that are not immediately needed for energy are stored in adipose tissue (fat cells) for later use. This storage is essential for maintaining energy reserves and providing insulation and protection for organs.

- **Mobilization:** When the body requires energy, such as during periods of fasting or physical activity, stored fats are mobilized. Hormones like adrenaline and glucagon signal adipose tissue to release fatty acids into the bloodstream through a process called lipolysis.
- **Transport in Bloodstream:** Fatty acids released from adipose tissue bind to carrier proteins (such as albumin) in the bloodstream for transport to tissues like muscle and liver.
- **Oxidation for Energy:** Fatty acids can be oxidized (broken down) in the mitochondria of cells to produce energy through a process called beta-oxidation. This process generates adenosine triphosphate (ATP), the body's primary energy currency.
- **Ketogenesis:** During prolonged periods of fasting or low carbohydrate intake, the liver converts fatty acids into ketone bodies through a process called ketogenesis. Ketone bodies can serve as an alternative fuel source for tissues, including the brain, when glucose availability is limited.
- **Regulation:** Fat metabolism is tightly regulated by various hormones and enzymes to maintain energy balance and meet the body's metabolic demands. Hormones such as insulin, glucagon, adrenaline, and leptin play key roles in regulating lipid metabolism by

influencing processes like lipolysis, lipogenesis, and fatty acid oxidation.

- **Synthesis:** In addition to dietary fats, the body can also synthesize fats de novo from other nutrients such as carbohydrates and proteins through a process called lipogenesis. This occurs primarily in the liver and adipose tissue and is influenced by factors like dietary intake, hormonal signaling, and metabolic status.

*Overall, **fat metabolism** is a complex and dynamic process that plays a critical role in energy homeostasis, nutrient storage, and cellular function throughout the body. Dysfunction in lipid metabolism can lead to various metabolic disorders such as obesity, diabetes, and cardiovascular diseases. Understanding the science behind fat metabolism is essential for developing strategies to maintain optimal health and prevent metabolic imbalances.*

ENERGY BALANCE: CALORIES IN VS. CALORIES OUT

Energy balance refers to the relationship between the calories you consume through food and beverages (calories in) and the calories you expend through physical activity and bodily functions (calories out). It is a fundamental concept in understanding weight management and overall health.

1. **Calories In (Consumption):** This refers to the number of calories you take in through the food and drinks you consume. Each food item has a certain number of calories, which represent the amount of energy it provides your body when metabolized. For example, a slice of bread might have around 100 calories, while a chocolate bar might have 200 calories.

2. **Calories Out (Expenditure):** Calories out encompasses various ways your body uses energy:

- *Basal Metabolic Rate (BMR): This is the amount of energy your body needs to maintain basic physiological functions like breathing, circulating blood, and cell production while at rest. BMR accounts for the largest portion of calories expended daily.*
- *Physical Activity: Any movement you do throughout the day, from walking to intense workouts, requires energy and contributes to calorie expenditure.*

- ***Thermic Effect of Food (TEF):*** *This is the energy expended during digestion, absorption, and metabolism of nutrients from food. Different macronutrients (carbohydrates, proteins, and fats) require varying amounts of energy to be metabolized.*
- ***Non-Exercise Activity Thermogenesis (NEAT):*** *This includes all the energy expended for activities that are not sleeping, eating, or sports-like exercise. It includes activities such as walking to work, typing, gardening, and fidgeting.*
- ***Adaptive Thermogenesis:*** *This is the adjustment of calorie expenditure in response to changes in diet and environmental conditions.*

If you consume more calories than you expend, you're in a state of positive energy balance, and your body stores the excess energy primarily as fat, leading to weight gain over time. Conversely, if you expend more calories than you consume, you're in a state of negative energy balance, and your body taps into its fat stores for energy, leading to weight loss.

Achieving and maintaining a healthy weight involves balancing calorie intake and expenditure. This can be done by adjusting your diet to include nutritious foods in appropriate portions and incorporating regular physical activity into your lifestyle.

2. NOURISHING YOUR BODY

Nutrition plays a pivotal role in weight management, influencing both the quantity and quality of food intake, as well as how the body utilizes nutrients for energy and other metabolic processes. Here are several key aspects of nutrition in weight management:

- **Caloric Balance:** Weight management fundamentally revolves around the balance between calories consumed and calories expended. If you consume more calories than your body needs for energy expenditure, you will gain weight. Conversely, if you consume fewer calories than you expend, you will lose weight. Therefore, understanding the caloric content of foods and controlling portion sizes is essential.
- **Macronutrient Composition:** The three macronutrients—carbohydrates, proteins, and fats—each play unique roles in weight management. Carbohydrates are the body's primary energy source, while proteins are crucial for muscle repair and maintenance. Fats provide energy and support various bodily functions. The proportion of these macronutrients in the diet can influence satiety, energy levels, and metabolic rate, all of which impact weight management.

- **Nutrient Density:** Choosing nutrient-dense foods—those that provide a high concentration of essential nutrients relative to their calorie content—supports overall health and can facilitate weight management. Foods rich in vitamins, minerals, fiber, and antioxidants are typically lower in calories and more satisfying, helping to control appetite and prevent overeating.
- **Hydration:** Adequate hydration is essential for overall health and can also influence weight management. Drinking water before meals can help reduce calorie intake by promoting feelings of fullness. Additionally, staying hydrated supports proper metabolism and can enhance exercise performance, which contributes to calorie expenditure.
- **Meal Timing and Frequency:** The timing and frequency of meals can impact weight management outcomes. Some evidence suggests that spreading calorie intake across multiple smaller meals throughout the day may help control hunger and stabilize blood sugar levels, while others find intermittent fasting or time-restricted eating patterns to be effective for weight loss. Ultimately, the best approach may vary based on individual preferences and lifestyle factors.

- **Behavioral and Psychological Factors:** Nutrition is closely intertwined with behavior and psychology when it comes to weight management. Emotional eating, stress, social influences, and environmental cues all play significant roles in food choices and eating habits.
- **Individual Variability:** It's important to recognize that there is no one-size-fits-all approach to nutrition and weight management. Factors such as age, gender, genetics, metabolism, activity level, and underlying health conditions can all influence nutrient needs and weight loss outcomes.

UNDERSTANDING MACRONUTRIENTS AND MICRONUTRIENTS

Macronutrients are nutrients that are required by the body in relatively large amounts to provide energy and support various bodily functions. There are three primary macronutrients:

1. **Carbohydrates:** Carbohydrates are the body's primary source of energy. They are found in foods like grains, fruits, vegetables, and legumes. Carbohydrates are broken down into glucose, which is used by the body for energy production.

2. **Proteins**: Proteins are crucial for building and repairing tissues, as well as for various metabolic processes. They are composed of amino acids, some of which are essential and must be obtained from the diet. Good sources of protein include meat, poultry, fish, eggs, dairy products, legumes, nuts, and seeds.

3. **Fats:** Fats are also important sources of energy and play a role in hormone production, cell membrane structure, and nutrient absorption. They are found in foods like oils, butter, nuts, seeds, avocados, and fatty fish. Fats are categorized into saturated fats, unsaturated fats, and trans fats, with unsaturated fats being considered the healthiest option.

Micronutrients are essential nutrients required by the body in smaller quantities for various physiological functions. They include vitamins and minerals:

1. **Vitamins:** Vitamins are organic compounds that are essential for normal growth and development, immune function, and overall health. There are two types of vitamins: fat-soluble vitamins (A, D, E, and K) and water-soluble vitamins (B vitamins and vitamin C). Each vitamin has specific functions and can be found in a variety of foods, including fruits, vegetables, grains, dairy products, and meats.

2. **Minerals:** Minerals are inorganic nutrients that are essential for various bodily functions, including bone health, nerve function, fluid balance, and energy production. Some important minerals include calcium, iron, magnesium, potassium, sodium, zinc, and selenium. These minerals can be obtained from a diverse range of foods, including fruits, vegetables, whole grains, dairy products, nuts, seeds, and lean meats.

Key Differences:

- Macronutrients provide energy (calories) to the body, whereas micronutrients do not provide energy directly but are essential for numerous metabolic processes.
- Macronutrients are required in larger quantities compared to micronutrients.
- Both macronutrients and micronutrients are necessary for overall health, and deficiencies in either can lead to various health problems.

STRATEGIES FOR MINDFUL EATING

Mindful eating involves paying full attention to the experience of eating and drinking, both internally and externally. It encourages being present in the moment, acknowledging physical and emotional sensations, and making conscious choices about food. Here's a breakdown of strategies for practicing mindful eating:

- **Engage All Senses:** Use sight, smell, touch, and even sound to fully engage with your food before taking a bite. Notice the colors, textures, and aromas. Appreciate the effort that went into preparing the meal.
- **Eat Slowly:** Take your time with each bite, savoring the flavors and textures. Chew your food thoroughly and put your utensils down between bites. Eating slowly helps you tune in to your body's hunger and fullness signals.
- **Listen to Your Body**: Pay attention to physical hunger cues like stomach growling, fatigue, or light-headedness. Also, be aware of emotional triggers for eating, such as stress or boredom. Before eating, ask yourself if you're truly hungry or if there's another need you're trying to fulfill.
- **Practice Gratitude**: Before you begin eating, take a moment to express gratitude for the food in front of you. Reflect on where it came from and the effort that went into producing it. Cultivating gratitude can enhance the enjoyment of your meal.

- **Mindful Portioning**: Serve yourself appropriate portions and pay attention to how much you're eating. Use smaller plates and bowls to help control portion sizes. Be mindful of portion distortion, where oversized servings can lead to overeating.

- **Eliminate Distractions**: Minimize distractions while eating, such as watching TV, scrolling through your phone, or working at your desk. Focus solely on the act of eating and the sensations it evokes.

- **Check-in with Hunger and Fullness:** Pause halfway through your meal to assess your hunger level. Are you still hungry, or are you satisfied? Aim to stop eating when you're comfortably full, rather than stuffed.

- **Non-Judgmental Awareness**: Approach your eating experiences with curiosity and non-judgment. Avoid labeling foods as "good" or "bad" and refrain from criticizing yourself for what or how much you're eating.

- **Slow Down:** Eating slowly allows your brain to catch up with your stomach, giving you a better sense of satiety. Put your fork down between bites, take deep breaths, and enjoy the experience of eating.

- **Reflect on Food Choices**: After finishing your meal, reflect on how the food made you feel physically and emotionally. Notice any patterns or tendencies in your eating habits without judgment, and consider how you might adjust your choices in the future.

- **Practice Mindful Eating Regularly:** Like any skill, mindful eating improves with practice. Aim to incorporate mindful eating into your routine regularly, whether it's for one meal a day or more. Over time, it will become more natural and intuitive.

3. MOVING TOWARDS MOVEMENT

Physical activity is a cornerstone of successful weight loss because it helps create a calorie deficit, boosts metabolism, preserves lean muscle mass, improves insulin sensitivity, enhances mental well-being, promotes a sustainable lifestyle change, and reduces the risk of chronic diseases. Combining regular exercise with a balanced diet is the most effective approach to achieving and maintaining a healthy weight. Physical activity plays a crucial role in weight loss for several reasons:

- **Calorie Burn:** When you engage in physical activity, your body burns calories for energy. The more intense the activity, the more calories you burn. By burning more calories than you consume through food and beverages, you create a calorie deficit, which is essential for weight loss.
- **Boosts Metabolism:** Regular physical activity can increase your metabolic rate, which is the rate at which your body burns calories at rest. This means that even when you're not exercising, you'll still be burning more calories throughout the day if you're physically active.
- **Preserves Lean Muscle Mass**: During weight loss, it's common for people to lose not only fat but also muscle mass. However, incorporating strength training or

resistance exercises into your routine can help preserve lean muscle mass. Muscle tissue is metabolically active, meaning it burns more calories than fat tissue, even at rest.

- **Improves Insulin Sensitivity:** Regular physical activity can improve insulin sensitivity, which is crucial for regulating blood sugar levels. When your body becomes more sensitive to insulin, it can more effectively remove glucose from the bloodstream and use it for energy rather than storing it as fat. Improved insulin sensitivity can also help prevent type 2 diabetes and other metabolic disorders.

- **Enhances Mental Well-being:** Exercise is not only beneficial for your physical health but also your mental health. Physical activity releases endorphins, which are neurotransmitters that promote feelings of happiness and reduce stress and anxiety. When you feel good mentally, you're more likely to stick to your weight loss goals and make healthier choices overall.

- **Lifestyle Change**: Incorporating regular physical activity into your routine promotes a sustainable lifestyle change rather than relying solely on restrictive diets. Exercise can become a habit that you enjoy and look forward to, making it easier to maintain your weight loss results in the long term.

- **Reduces Risk of Chronic Diseases**: Being overweight or obese is associated with an increased risk of several chronic diseases, including heart disease, stroke, type 2 diabetes, certain cancers, and more. By losing weight through physical activity and maintaining a healthy weight, you can lower your risk of developing these conditions and improve overall health and longevity.
- **Appetite Regulation:** Regular physical activity can help regulate appetite hormones, such as ghrelin and leptin. Exercise can decrease levels of ghrelin, the hormone responsible for stimulating hunger, and increase levels of leptin, the hormone that signals feelings of fullness.
- **Improved Sleep Quality:** Physical activity has been linked to improved sleep quality. Getting an adequate amount of quality sleep is essential for weight loss and overall health. Poor sleep can disrupt appetite-regulating hormones, increase cravings for unhealthy foods, and negatively impact metabolism. Regular exercise can help promote better sleep patterns, which can indirectly support weight loss efforts.
- **Increased Energy Levels**: This can lead to greater motivation to stay active throughout the day and participate in other activities that support weight loss, such as meal preparation and planning.

FINDING JOY IN EXERCISE: FROM WALKING TO WEIGHTLIFTING

Finding joy in exercise encompasses a spectrum of activities, from the simple pleasure of walking to the more intense and focused discipline of weightlifting. Here's how these activities contribute to joy and well-being:

- **Walking:** Walking is one of the most accessible forms of exercise. It requires no special equipment, can be done almost anywhere, and is gentle on the body. Finding joy in walking often comes from the opportunity it provides to connect with nature, clear one's mind, and engage in mindful movement. Whether it's a leisurely stroll through a park or a brisk walk along a scenic trail, walking allows individuals to appreciate their surroundings, breathe fresh air, and experience a sense of freedom and rejuvenation.
- **Running**: Similar to walking, running offers a chance to experience the outdoors and enjoy the benefits of cardiovascular exercise. Many people find joy in the rhythmic motion of running, the release of endorphins (often referred to as "runner's high"), and the sense of accomplishment that comes with reaching new distances or speed goals. Running can also be a social activity, as people often join running groups or participate in races, fostering a sense of community and camaraderie.

- **Cycling:** Cycling combines physical activity with the pleasure of exploration and adventure. Whether it's cycling through scenic countryside, navigating urban streets, or participating in group rides, cycling offers a sense of freedom and exhilaration. Many people find joy in the feeling of speed, the wind against their face, and the opportunity to discover new places while getting fit.
- **Swimming:** Swimming provides a full-body workout while being low-impact on the joints. For many, the sensation of being in the water is calming and meditative, allowing them to focus on their strokes and breathing. Whether it's swimming laps in a pool, enjoying the tranquility of a natural body of water, or participating in water-based activities like water aerobics or snorkeling, swimming offers both physical and mental benefits that contribute to joy and well-being.
- **Weightlifting:** While weightlifting may seem intimidating to some, many people find joy in the challenge and sense of empowerment it provides. Strength training not only builds muscle and improves physical health but also enhances confidence and resilience. Setting and achieving strength goals, feeling the progression in lifting heavier weights, and experiencing the tangible results of strength gains can be incredibly rewarding.

- Additionally, weightlifting can foster a sense of discipline, focus, and mental toughness that carries over into other areas of life.

In summary, finding joy in exercise is about discovering activities that resonate with individual preferences, interests, and goals. Whether it's the simplicity of walking, the intensity of weightlifting, or anything in between, regular physical activity has the power to improve mood, boost energy levels, and enhance overall well-being. The key is to explore different forms of exercise, listen to your body, and prioritize activities that bring you happiness and fulfillment.

OVERCOMING BARRIERS TO STAYING ACTIVE

Overcoming barriers to staying active involves identifying and addressing obstacles that prevent individuals from engaging in regular physical activity. These barriers can be physical, psychological, social, or environmental in nature. Here are some strategies to overcome these barriers:

- **Time constraints:** Many people cite lack of time as a barrier to exercise. To overcome this, prioritize physical activity by scheduling it into your daily routine. Break it down into smaller sessions if needed, and choose activities that can easily fit into your schedule, such as brisk walking during lunch breaks or taking the stairs instead of the elevator.
- **Lack of motivation:** Find activities that you enjoy and that align with your interests and goals. Set realistic and achievable goals to keep yourself motivated. Additionally, exercising with a friend or joining group classes can provide social support and accountability, making it more enjoyable and motivating.
- **Environmental barriers:** Identify environmental factors that may hinder your ability to stay active, such as lack of access to safe exercise facilities, inclement weather, or neighborhood safety concerns. Look for alternative indoor activities or home-based workouts during unfavorable weather conditions.

- **Financial constraints**: Staying active doesn't necessarily require expensive gym memberships or equipment. Look for low-cost or free exercise options, such as walking or jogging in local parks, utilizing community recreation centers, or following online workout videos. (***Buy our book 3 for Workouts suitable for Weight Loss***)
- **Lack of knowledge or skills:** If you're unsure about how to start or maintain a physical activity routine, seek out resources and information to educate yourself.
- **Psychological barriers:** Address any psychological barriers such as fear of judgment, low self-confidence, or stress. Practice self-compassion and focus on the positive aspects of physical activity, such as improved mood, energy levels, and overall well-being. Engage in stress-reducing activities like yoga, meditation, or deep breathing exercises to help manage psychological barriers to staying active.

By identifying and addressing these barriers, individuals can develop strategies to overcome obstacles and establish a sustainable and enjoyable physical activity routine that promotes health and well-being. Remember that consistency and perseverance are key to long-term success in staying active.

INCORPORATING MOVEMENT INTO YOUR DAILY LIFE

Incorporating movement into your daily life involves intentionally integrating physical activity into your routine, beyond dedicated exercise sessions. It's about embracing a lifestyle that prioritizes movement throughout your day, rather than viewing exercise as a separate task.

Here are some ways to incorporate movement into your daily life:

- **Active Commuting:** Instead of driving everywhere, consider walking, biking, or using public transportation. This adds movement to your day while reducing carbon emissions and saving money.
- **Take Breaks:** Whether you work at a desk or are at home, take regular breaks to stand up, stretch, or take a short walk. This not only helps prevent stiffness and muscle fatigue but also boosts productivity and creativity.
- **Use Stairs:** Opt for stairs instead of elevators or escalators whenever possible. Climbing stairs is an excellent way to engage multiple muscle groups and increase cardiovascular health.
- **Active Hobbies:** Choose hobbies that involve physical activity, such as gardening, dancing, hiking, or playing a sport. This makes staying active feel enjoyable rather than a chore.

- **Household Chores:** Turn everyday tasks into opportunities for movement. Cleaning, gardening, cooking, and doing laundry all require physical effort and can contribute to your daily activity level.
- **Walk and Talk:** Instead of sitting down for phone calls or meetings, walk while you talk. This can be done indoors or outdoors and adds steps to your day without requiring extra time.
- **Stand Up:** If you have a sedentary job, consider using a standing desk or incorporating standing breaks throughout the day. Standing engages your muscles and can help alleviate back pain associated with prolonged sitting.
- **Active Socializing:** Instead of meeting friends for coffee or drinks, suggest activities like hiking, biking, or playing a sport together. This allows you to catch up while also staying active.
- **Scheduled Movement:** Set reminders on your phone or calendar to prompt you to move throughout the day. Even short bursts of activity can have significant health benefits.
- **Mindful Movement:** Incorporate mindfulness practices like yoga or tai chi into your routine. These activities not only promote physical health but also reduce stress and improve mental well-being.

4. MASTERING MINDSET

The psychology of weight loss, particularly in overcoming emotional eating, delves into the complex relationship between our emotions, behaviors, and eating habits. Emotional eating refers to the tendency to eat in response to emotions rather than physical hunger. This can include eating to soothe stress, cope with sadness, celebrate happiness, or even out of boredom. Overcoming emotional eating is a critical aspect of successful weight loss because it addresses the root causes of unhealthy eating patterns. Several psychological factors contribute to emotional eating:

- **Emotional Triggers:** Emotional eating often stems from specific triggers such as stress, anxiety, depression, loneliness, or boredom. Individuals may turn to food as a way to numb uncomfortable emotions or seek comfort.
- **Learned Behavior:** Many people learn to associate certain emotions with eating from a young age. For example, receiving food as a reward or comfort during childhood can create lasting patterns of emotional eating.
- **Social and Environmental Influences:** Social and environmental factors, such as cultural norms, family dynamics, and advertising, can influence eating behaviors and attitudes toward food.

- Emotional eating may be reinforced by societal messages that promote food as a source of comfort or reward.
- **Biological Factors:** Hormonal fluctuations, neurotransmitter imbalances, and genetic predispositions can also play a role in emotional eating. For instance, stress can trigger the release of cortisol, which may increase cravings for high-calorie foods.
- To overcome emotional eating and achieve sustainable weight loss, individuals can implement various psychological strategies:
- **Mindfulness:** Practicing mindfulness techniques, such as mindful eating, helps individuals become more aware of their emotions, thoughts, and physical sensations related to eating. By paying attention to hunger cues and eating mindfully, individuals can break the cycle of emotional eating.
- **Emotion Regulation:** Learning healthy ways to cope with emotions is essential for overcoming emotional eating. This may involve developing alternative coping strategies such as journaling, deep breathing exercises, practicing relaxation techniques, or seeking support from friends, family, or a therapist.

- **Identifying Triggers:** Understanding the specific emotions and situations that trigger emotional eating is key to developing targeted strategies for managing cravings. Keeping a food diary or journal can help individuals identify patterns and triggers related to emotional eating.

- **Building a Support System:** Surrounding oneself with supportive friends, family members, or a support group can provide encouragement, accountability, and practical advice for overcoming emotional eating and achieving weight loss goals.

- **Cognitive Behavioral Therapy (CBT):** CBT is a therapeutic approach that helps individuals identify and challenge negative thought patterns and behaviors. It can be effective in treating emotional eating by addressing underlying beliefs and promoting healthier coping strategies.

- **Healthy Lifestyle Habits:** Establishing regular meal times, prioritizing nutritious foods, staying physically active, getting adequate sleep, and managing stress are all important components of a healthy lifestyle that can support weight loss and reduce the likelihood of emotional eating.

CULTIVATING SELF-COMPASSION AND RESILIENCE

Cultivating self-compassion and resilience involves developing a mindset and set of practices that enable individuals to navigate life's challenges with greater emotional strength and well-being.

- **Self-Compassion:** This refers to treating oneself with kindness, understanding, and acceptance, particularly in the face of failure, setbacks, or suffering. Instead of harsh self-criticism or judgment, self-compassionate individuals acknowledge their pain or mistakes with a sense of warmth and understanding, recognizing that imperfection and difficulties are part of the human experience. Self-compassion involves three main components:
    a. **Self-Kindness:** Being gentle and understanding toward oneself rather than harshly critical or self-judgmental.
    b. **Common Humanity:** Recognizing that suffering and setbacks are a normal part of the human condition, understanding that everyone experiences them at some point.
    c. **Mindfulness:** Being aware of one's thoughts and emotions without getting overly absorbed or identified with them.

Resilience: Resilience refers to the ability to bounce back from adversity, adapt to change, and cope effectively with stress. Resilient individuals are not immune to hardship, but they possess certain qualities and skills that help them navigate challenges more effectively. These might include:

- **Positive Outlook:** Maintaining a hopeful and optimistic attitude, even in the face of adversity, which helps to sustain motivation and perseverance.
- **Problem-Solving Skills:** Being able to identify and implement effective solutions to problems, rather than feeling overwhelmed or helpless in the face of difficulties.
- **Social Support:** Having a strong network of supportive relationships, whether with friends, family, or community, which provides emotional support and practical assistance during tough times.
- **Adaptability:** Being flexible and open to change, able to adjust one's goals, plans, and strategies in response to new circumstances or challenges.

Combining self-compassion and resilience involves applying self-compassionate principles and practices to build resilience and emotional strength.

SETTING REALISTIC GOALS AND CELEBRATING PROGRESS

Setting realistic goals involves establishing objectives that are achievable within a certain timeframe and with the available resources. It's important because realistic goals are more likely to be accomplished, boosting motivation and morale. When setting goals, it's crucial to consider factors such as one's capabilities, limitations, and the external environment.

Celebrating progress involves acknowledging and rewarding achievements made towards those goals, regardless of how small they may seem. This can take various forms, such as verbal recognition, treats, or other forms of self-reward. Celebrating progress is vital because it reinforces positive behaviors, sustains motivation, and provides a sense of accomplishment.

Here's a breakdown of the importance and benefits of both:

Setting Realistic Goals:

- **Achievability**: Realistic goals are within reach based on current resources, skills, and circumstances. They provide a clear path forward without overwhelming or demotivating individuals.
- **Clarity**: Realistic goals help in defining clear objectives and understanding what needs to be done to achieve them.

- **Motivation:** Goals that are achievable create a sense of purpose and motivation to work towards them. When people believe they can accomplish something, they are more likely to put in the effort required.
- **Measurement:** Realistic goals are measurable, making it easier to track progress and make adjustments as necessary.
- **Sustainability:** Setting realistic goals helps prevent burnout by avoiding setting unattainable targets that lead to frustration and disappointment.

Celebrating Progress:
- **Motivation:** Celebrating progress reinforces positive behavior and boosts motivation. It provides a sense of accomplishment, encouraging individuals to keep working towards their goals.
- **Recognition:** Celebrating progress acknowledges the effort and dedication put into achieving goals. This recognition can be a powerful morale booster and increase engagement.
- **Feedback Loop:** Celebrating progress allows individuals to reflect on what they've accomplished and learn from their experiences. It provides valuable feedback that can inform future actions and goal-setting.

- **Sustained Momentum:** By acknowledging progress, individuals are more likely to maintain momentum and continue striving for success. It prevents stagnation and encourages continuous improvement.
- **Sense of Satisfaction:** Celebrating progress cultivates a sense of satisfaction and fulfillment, contributing to overall well-being and happiness.

SKINNY BUFFALO CHICKEN DIP

PREP 10 Mins	**COOK** 25 Mins	**SERVING SIZE** 8	**POINTS** 0

INGREDIENTS

- 2 cups cooked chicken breast, shredded
- 1/2 cup plain non-fat Greek yogurt
- 1/2 cup Frank's RedHot Original Cayenne Pepper Sauce (or any buffalo hot sauce)
- 1/4 cup fat-free cream cheese, softened
- 1/4 cup fat-free mayonnaise
- 1/4 cup crumbled fat-free feta cheese (optional)
- 1/4 cup chopped green onions (optional)
- 1/4 teaspoon garlic powder
- 1/4 teaspoon onion powder
- Salt and pepper to taste
- Cooking spray

DIRECTIONS

- Preheat your oven to 350°F (175°C).
- In a large mixing bowl, combine the shredded chicken, Greek yogurt, hot sauce, cream cheese, mayonnaise, feta cheese (if using), green onions (if using), garlic powder, onion powder, salt, and pepper. Mix well until everything is evenly combined.
- Lightly coat a baking dish with cooking spray to prevent sticking.
- Transfer the chicken mixture into the prepared baking dish, spreading it out evenly.
- Bake in the preheated oven for about 20-25 minutes or until the dip is heated through and bubbly around the edges.
- Once done, remove from the oven and let it cool for a few minutes before serving.

TURKEY CHILI

PREP	**COOK**	**SERVING SIZE**	**POINTS**
10 Mins	25 Mins	1/2	2

INGREDIENTS

- 1/2 teaspoon olive oil
- 1/4 cup onion, diced
- 1/4 cup red bell pepper, diced
- 4 ounces lean ground turkey
- 1 clove garlic, minced
- 1/2 can (7.25 ounces) diced tomatoes, undrained
- 1/2 can (7.75 ounces) kidney beans, drained and rinsed
- 1/2 tablespoon chili powder
- 1/2 teaspoon cumin
- Salt and pepper to taste
- Optional toppings: chopped fresh cilantro, diced avocado, low-fat shredded cheese, non-fat Greek yogurt

DIRECTIONS

- Heat olive oil in a pot, then sauté diced onion and red bell pepper until softened.
- Add lean ground turkey, cooking until browned, and stir in minced garlic.
- Pour in half of the diced tomatoes and half of the kidney beans.
- Season with half of the chili powder and half of the cumin, plus salt and pepper to taste.
- Simmer the chili for 15-20 minutes, stirring occasionally.
- Taste and adjust seasoning if necessary.
- Serve hot, optionally topped with cilantro, avocado, cheese, or yogurt.

GRILLED SHRIMP TACOS

PREP
15 Mins

COOK
10 Mins

SERVING SIZE
2

POINTS
3

INGREDIENTS

- 12 large shrimp, peeled and deveined
- 1 teaspoon olive oil (5 sprays from a cooking spray bottle)
- 1 teaspoon chili powder
- 1/2 teaspoon cumin
- Salt and pepper to taste
- 6 small corn tortillas (each tortilla about 1.5 points)
- 1 cup shredded lettuce
- 1/2 cup diced tomatoes
- 1/4 cup diced red onion
- 1/4 cup chopped cilantro
- 2 tablespoons plain non-fat Greek yogurt
- 2 tablespoons salsa (choose a low-point or zero-point option)
- Lime wedges for serving

DIRECTIONS

- Preheat your grill to medium-high heat.
- Toss shrimp with chili powder, cumin, salt, and pepper. Grill for 2-3 minutes per side.
- Heat tortillas on the grill for 30 seconds per side.
- Divide lettuce, tomatoes, onion, and cilantro among tortillas. Add grilled shrimp.
- Drizzle each taco with 1 tbsp of Greek yogurt and 1 tbsp of salsa.
- Serve immediately with lime wedges on the side.

LIGHTENED-UP MAC AND CHEESE

PREP
15 Mins

COOK
25 Mins

SERVING SIZE
6

POINTS
7

INGREDIENTS

- 8 oz (about 2 cups) whole wheat elbow macaroni
- 2 cups cauliflower florets
- 1 cup low-fat milk
- 1 cup shredded reduced-fat cheddar cheese
- 1/4 cup grated Parmesan cheese
- 1/2 teaspoon garlic powder
- 1/2 teaspoon onion powder
- Salt and pepper to taste
- Cooking spray

DIRECTIONS

- Cook macaroni according to package instructions. Drain and set aside.
- Boil cauliflower until tender, about 5-7 minutes. Drain and set aside.
- In a pot, heat milk until warm. Stir in cheddar and Parmesan until melted and smooth.
- Add cauliflower, garlic powder, onion powder, salt, and pepper to cheese sauce. Stir.
- Combine macaroni with cheese sauce mixture.
- Transfer to a baking dish sprayed with cooking spray.
- Bake at 375°F (190°C) for 20-25 minutes, until bubbly and golden.
- Serve hot.

CAULIFLOWER PIZZA CRUST

PREP 15 Mins	**COOK** 40 Mins	**SERVING SIZE** 4	**POINTS** 4

INGREDIENTS

- 1 medium head cauliflower, cut into florets
- 1/4 cup grated Parmesan cheese
- 1/4 cup reduced-fat mozzarella cheese
- 1/4 teaspoon dried oregano
- 1/4 teaspoon garlic powder
- 1/4 teaspoon salt
- 1/4 teaspoon black pepper
- 1 egg, lightly beaten

DIRECTIONS

- Preheat oven to 400°F (200°C) and line a baking sheet with parchment paper.
- Pulse cauliflower florets in a food processor until they resemble rice.
- Microwave riced cauliflower for 4-5 minutes, then let it cool.
- Squeeze out moisture from the cooled cauliflower using a kitchen towel.
- Mix cauliflower with cheeses, spices, and egg in a bowl.
- Spread mixture onto the prepared baking sheet to form a crust.
- Bake for 20-25 minutes until golden brown.
- Add desired toppings, then bake for another 10-15 minutes.
- Slice and serve hot.

BBQ CHICKEN FLATBREAD PIZZA

PREP 10 Mins	**COOK** 12 Mins	**SERVING SIZE** 1/2	**POINTS** 4

INGREDIENTS

- 2 whole wheat flatbreads (such as Flatout Light)
- 1/2 cup BBQ sauce (look for a lower sugar option to keep points lower)
- 1 cup cooked, shredded chicken breast
- 1/2 cup diced red onion
- 1/2 cup diced bell peppers (any color)
- 1 cup shredded reduced-fat mozzarella cheese
- Fresh cilantro, chopped (optional)
- Salt and pepper to taste

DIRECTIONS

- Preheat oven to 375°F (190°C).
- Place flatbreads on baking sheet.
- Spread BBQ sauce on each.
- Top with chicken, onions, bell peppers, cheese.
- Season with salt and pepper.
- Bake for 10-12 minutes.
- Let cool briefly.
- Optional: sprinkle with cilantro.
- Slice each into 4 pieces.
- Serve.

GREEK YOGURT RANCH DRESSING

PREP	COOK	SERVING SIZE	POINTS
10 Mins	0 Mins	2	4

INGREDIENTS

- 1 cup non-fat Greek yogurt
- 1 tablespoon chopped fresh chives
- 1 tablespoon chopped fresh parsley
- 1 tablespoon chopped fresh dill
- 1 clove garlic, minced
- 1 teaspoon onion powder
- 1 teaspoon dried dill
- 1 teaspoon dried parsley
- 1 teaspoon dried chives
- 1/2 teaspoon salt
- 1/4 teaspoon black pepper
- 2 tablespoons skim milk (optional, for thinning)

DIRECTIONS

- In a mixing bowl, combine the Greek yogurt, fresh chives, fresh parsley, fresh dill, minced garlic, onion powder, dried dill, dried parsley, dried chives, salt, and black pepper.
- Mix well until all ingredients are thoroughly combined. If the dressing is too thick for your liking, you can add skim milk gradually until you reach your desired consistency.
- Taste and adjust seasoning if necessary.
- Transfer the dressing to a serving container or jar with a tight-fitting lid.
- Refrigerate for at least 30 minutes before serving to allow the flavors to meld together.
- Serve with your favorite salads or vegetables.

BLACK BEAN QUINOA SALAD

PREP
15 Mins

COOK
20 Mins

SERVING SIZE
6

POINTS
6

INGREDIENTS

- 3/4 cup dry quinoa
- 1 can (15 ounces) black beans, drained and rinsed
- 3/4 cup corn kernels (fresh, canned, or frozen)
- 1/2 bell pepper, diced
- 1/4 red onion, finely chopped
- 2 tablespoons fresh cilantro, chopped
- 1/2 avocado, diced
- Juice of 1 lime
- 1 tablespoon olive oil
- 1/2 teaspoon ground cumin
- Salt and pepper to taste

DIRECTIONS

- Rinse 3/4 cup quinoa, then cook with 1 1/2 cups water until tender and water is absorbed.
- Combine cooked quinoa, black beans, corn, bell pepper, onion, and cilantro in a bowl.
- Whisk lime juice, olive oil, cumin, salt, and pepper in a small bowl.
- Pour dressing over salad, toss to coat.
- Gently fold in diced avocado.
- Chill if desired, then serve.

RATATOUILLE

PREP	COOK	SERVING SIZE	POINTS
15 Mins	25 Mins	6	0

INGREDIENTS

- 1 medium eggplant, diced
- 2 medium zucchinis, diced
- 1 large onion, diced
- 1 red bell pepper, diced
- 1 yellow bell pepper, diced
- 2 cloves garlic, minced
- 2 cups diced tomatoes (fresh or canned)
- 1 tablespoon tomato paste (optional)
- 1 teaspoon dried thyme
- 1 teaspoon dried oregano
- Salt and pepper to taste
- Cooking spray

DIRECTIONS

- Preheat oven to 400°F (200°C) and spray a baking dish with cooking spray.
- Combine diced vegetables and garlic in a large bowl.
- Mix diced tomatoes, tomato paste, thyme, oregano, salt, and pepper in a small bowl.
- Pour tomato mixture over vegetables and toss to coat.
- Transfer mixture to baking dish, spread evenly.
- Cover with foil and bake for 20 minutes.
- Remove foil and bake for another 5-10 minutes until tender.
- Serve and enjoy!

GRILLED MEDITERRANEAN CHICKEN SKEWERS

PREP 15 Mins	**COOK** 12 Mins	**SERVING SIZE** 1	**POINTS** 1

INGREDIENTS

- 1 boneless, skinless chicken breast (4 oz)
- 1/4 cup cherry tomatoes
- 1/4 cup red onion, chopped into chunks
- 1/4 cup bell peppers, chopped into chunks (any color you prefer)
- 1 tablespoon olive oil
- 1 clove garlic, minced
- 1 tablespoon lemon juice
- 1/2 teaspoon dried oregano
- Salt and pepper to taste
- Wooden skewers, soaked in water for 30 minutes to prevent burning

DIRECTIONS

- Cut chicken into 1-inch chunks and marinate with olive oil, garlic, lemon juice, oregano, salt, and pepper.
- Chop vegetables into chunks.
- Preheat grill to medium-high heat.
- Thread chicken and vegetables onto soaked skewers.
- Grill skewers for 5-6 minutes on each side until chicken is cooked through and vegetables are tender.
- Let cool for a minute before serving.

ZUCCHINI NOODLES WITH PESTO

PREP
15 Mins

COOK
10 Mins

SERVING SIZE
4

POINTS
6

INGREDIENTS

- 4 medium zucchinis, spiralized into noodles
- 2 tablespoons olive oil
- 2 cloves garlic, minced
- 1/4 cup grated Parmesan cheese
- Salt and pepper to taste

Pesto:

- 2 cups fresh basil leaves
- 1/4 cup pine nuts
- 2 cloves garlic
- 1/4 cup grated Parmesan cheese
- 1/4 cup olive oil
- Salt and pepper to taste

DIRECTIONS

- In a food processor, combine basil leaves, pine nuts, garlic, and Parmesan cheese. Pulse until finely chopped.
- Make the pesto by blending basil, pine nuts, garlic, Parmesan, olive oil, salt, and pepper until smooth.
- Heat olive oil in a skillet, add minced garlic, and cook until fragrant.
- Add zucchini noodles to the skillet and toss to coat with garlic oil. Cook for 2-3 minutes until just tender.
- Remove skillet from heat and stir in prepared pesto until noodles are evenly coated.
- Season with salt and pepper, sprinkle with grated Parmesan
- Serve hot, garnished with additional Parmesan cheese and fresh basil if desired.

SPANISH GAZPACHO

PREP
15 Mins

COOK
0 Mins

SERVING SIZE
1

POINTS
3

INGREDIENTS

- 6 ripe tomatoes, chopped
- 1 cucumber, peeled and chopped
- 1 bell pepper, chopped (red or green)
- 1 small onion, chopped
- 2 cloves garlic, minced
- 2 tablespoons olive oil
- 2 tablespoons red wine vinegar
- 1 teaspoon salt
- 1/2 teaspoon black pepper
- 1/2 teaspoon cumin
- 1/4 teaspoon paprika
- 2 cups low-sodium tomato juice
- 1 tablespoon fresh lemon juice
- Optional toppings: diced avocado, croutons, chopped cilantro

DIRECTIONS

- In a blender or food processor, combine the chopped tomatoes, cucumber, bell pepper, onion, and garlic.
- Add olive oil, red wine vinegar, salt, black pepper, cumin, paprika, tomato juice, and lemon juice to the blender.
- Blend until smooth. You may need to do this in batches depending on the size of your blender.
- Taste and adjust seasoning if necessary.
- Refrigerate for at least 2 hours before serving to allow flavors to meld.
- Serve chilled with optional toppings if desired.

ITALIAN STUFFED BELL PEPPERS

PREP
15 Mins

COOK
35 Mins

SERVING
6

POINTS
3

INGREDIENTS

- 4 large bell peppers (any color)
- 1 pound lean ground turkey
- 1 small onion, diced
- 2 cloves garlic, minced
- 1 cup cooked brown rice
- 1 cup marinara sauce (look for a low-sugar, low-fat option)
- 1 teaspoon dried oregano
- 1 teaspoon dried basil
- Salt and pepper to taste
- Cooking spray

DIRECTIONS

- Preheat oven to 375°F (190°C).
- Cut tops off bell peppers, remove seeds and membranes.
- Sauté onion and garlic until translucent.
- Add ground turkey, cook until browned.
- Stir in rice, marinara sauce, oregano, basil, salt, and pepper. Cook for 2-3 minutes.
- Fill peppers with mixture, place in baking dish.
- Cover with foil, bake for 25-30 minutes.
- Optionally, add cheese and bake for additional 5 minutes.
- Serve hot.

GREEK LEMON CHICKEN SOUP

PREP	**COOK**	**SERVING SIZE**	**POINTS**
10 Mins	15 Mins	1 1/2	0

INGREDIENTS

- 4 cups fat-free chicken broth
- 1 cup water
- 1 cup cooked, shredded chicken breast (skinless, boneless)
- 1/2 cup uncooked orzo pasta
- 2 large eggs
- 1/4 cup fresh lemon juice
- Zest of 1 lemon
- 1/4 cup chopped fresh dill
- Salt and pepper to taste
- Optional: Lemon slices and additional dill for garnish.

DIRECTIONS

- Bring chicken broth and water to a boil in a large pot.
- Add orzo pasta, cook until al dente.
- In a bowl, whisk eggs, lemon juice, and zest.
- Slowly pour egg mixture into the pot, stirring constantly.
- Add shredded chicken, stir.
- Mix in chopped dill, salt, and pepper.
- Simmer for 2-3 minutes.
- Serve hot, garnish with lemon slices and dill.

FRENCH ONION SOUP

<table>
<tr><td>PREP
10 Mins</td><td>COOK
40 Mins</td><td>SERVING SIZE
2</td><td>POINTS
2</td></tr>
</table>

INGREDIENTS

- 4 large onions, thinly sliced
- 4 cups beef broth (low sodium, if possible)
- 1 tablespoon olive oil
- 1 teaspoon sugar
- 1 teaspoon balsamic vinegar
- Salt and pepper to taste
- 2 slices of whole-grain bread (or any bread of your choice)
- 1/4 cup shredded reduced-fat Swiss cheese

DIRECTIONS

- Heat oil, cook onions until caramelized (30-40 min).
- Sprinkle sugar over onions, cook for 5 more minutes.
- Add balsamic vinegar, scrape browned bits
- Pour in beef broth, simmer for 10 minutes. Season with salt and pepper.
- While soup simmers, preheat oven broiler.
- Ladle soup into oven-safe bowls. Top with bread slice, Swiss cheese.
- Place bowls under broiler until cheese melts (2-3 min).
- Carefully remove from oven, serve hot.

IRISH COLCANNON

PREP
15 Mins

COOK
25 Mins

SERVING SIZE
1/4

POINTS
4

INGREDIENTS

- 1 pound russet potatoes, peeled and diced
- 1/2 head green cabbage, thinly sliced
- 1 small onion, finely chopped
- 2 cloves garlic, minced
- 2 tablespoons reduced-fat butter or margarine
- 1/4 cup fat-free milk
- Salt and pepper to taste
- Optional: chopped scallions or parsley for garnish

DIRECTIONS

- Boil potatoes until tender, about 15-20 minutes. Drain.
- Steam or boil cabbage until tender, about 5-7 minutes. Drain.
- Sauté onion and garlic in butter until softened, about 3-5 minutes.
- Mash potatoes and cabbage with onion mixture.
- Stir in milk until desired consistency.
- Season with salt and pepper.
- Serve hot, garnished with scallions or parsley if desired.

SPINACH AND CHEESE QUICHE

PREP 15 Mins	**COOK** 40 Mins	**SERVING SIZE** 8	**POINTS** 7

INGREDIENTS

- 1 pre-made pie crust (whole wheat for a healthier option, ensure it's within your points allowance)
- 4 large eggs
- 1 cup unsweetened almond milk (or other non-dairy milk)
- 1 cup shredded reduced-fat cheese (such as cheddar or mozzarella)
- 2 cups chopped spinach (fresh or frozen, thawed and drained)
- 1/4 cup diced onions
- Salt and pepper to taste

DIRECTIONS

- Preheat your oven to 375°F (190°C).
- If using a frozen pie crust, allow it to thaw according to package instructions. If using a homemade crust, prepare it and place it in a pie dish.
- In a bowl, beat the eggs and almond milk together until well combined.
- Stir in the shredded cheese, chopped spinach, diced onions, salt, and pepper.
- Pour the egg mixture into the prepared pie crust.
- Bake in the preheated oven for 35-40 minutes, or until the quiche is set and the crust is golden brown.
- Remove from the oven and let it cool for a few minutes before slicing and serving.

WHOLE WHEAT PANCAKES

PREP	COOK	SERVING	POINTS
5 Mins	10 Mins	8	2

INGREDIENTS

- 1 cup whole wheat flour
- 1 tablespoon sugar (or sweetener of choice)
- 1 teaspoon baking powder
- 1/2 teaspoon baking soda
- 1/4 teaspoon salt
- 1 cup non-fat milk (or any milk of your choice)
- 1 large egg
- 1 tablespoon vegetable oil (or melted butter)
- Cooking spray or additional oil for greasing the pan

DIRECTIONS

- Mix dry ingredients: In a bowl, whisk flour, sugar, baking powder, baking soda, and salt.
- Combine wet ingredients: In another bowl, whisk milk, egg, and oil.
- Mix: Combine wet and dry ingredients until just combined.
- Preheat skillet: Heat skillet over medium heat and lightly grease.
- Cook pancakes: Pour 1/4 cup batter onto skillet per pancake.
- Flip: Cook until bubbles form, then flip and cook until golden brown.
- Repeat: Continue with remaining batter.
- Serve: Enjoy warm with desired toppings.

BUCKWHEAT PANCAKES

PREP
5 Mins

COOK
10 Mins

SERVING
8

POINTS
2

INGREDIENTS

- 1/4 cup buckwheat flour
- 1/4 teaspoon baking powder
- 1/4 cup unsweetened almond milk (or any milk of your choice)
- 1 egg white
- 1/4 teaspoon vanilla extract
- Non-stick cooking spray

DIRECTIONS

- Mix dry ingredients in one bowl and wet ingredients in another.
- Combine wet and dry ingredients.
- Heat skillet, coat with cooking spray.
- Pour 1/4 cup batter for each pancake.
- Cook until bubbles form (2-3 min), flip and cook until golden (1-2 min).
- Repeat with remaining batter.
- Serve warm with desired toppings.

MOCHA BANANA SMOOTHIE

PREP	COOK	SERVING
5 Mins	10 Mins	2

INGREDIENTS

- 1 ripe banana, frozen
- 1 cup brewed coffee, chilled
- 1/2 cup unsweetened almond milk
- 1 tablespoon unsweetened cocoa powder
- 1 tablespoon honey or maple syrup (optional, adjust according to taste)
- 1/2 teaspoon vanilla extract
- 1 cup ice cubes

DIRECTIONS

Preparation:
- Brew coffee ahead of time and let it chill in the refrigerator.
- Peel ripe banana, slice it, and freeze it for at least 2 hours.

Blend:
- In a blender, combine the frozen banana, chilled coffee, almond milk, cocoa powder, honey or maple syrup (if using), vanilla extract, and ice cubes.
- Blend until smooth and creamy, adjusting sweetness if necessary.

Serve:
- Pour the smoothie into glasses and serve immediately.

BUCKWHEAT PANCAKES

PREP	**COOK**	**SERVING**	**POINTS**
5 Mins	10 Mins	8	2

INGREDIENTS

- 1/4 cup buckwheat flour
- 1/4 teaspoon baking powder
- 1/4 cup unsweetened almond milk (or any milk of your choice)
- 1 egg white
- 1/4 teaspoon vanilla extract
- Non-stick cooking spray

DIRECTIONS

- Mix dry ingredients in one bowl and wet ingredients in another.
- Combine wet and dry ingredients.
- Heat skillet, coat with cooking spray.
- Pour 1/4 cup batter for each pancake.
- Cook until bubbles form (2-3 min), flip and cook until golden (1-2 min).
- Repeat with remaining batter.
- Serve warm with desired toppings.

EGGPLANT PARMESAN STACKS

PREP
10 Mins

COOK
20 Mins

SERVING
2

POINTS
2

INGREDIENTS

- 1 medium eggplant
- 1 cup marinara sauce (low-calorie)
- 1/2 cup shredded part-skim mozzarella cheese
- 2 tablespoons grated Parmesan cheese
- 1/4 cup breadcrumbs (whole wheat or seasoned)
- Cooking spray
- Salt and pepper to taste
- Optional: fresh basil leaves for garnish

DIRECTIONS

- Preheat oven to 400°F (200°C).
- Slice eggplant into 1/4-inch rounds and pat dry.
- Dip slices in breadcrumbs and place on a baking sheet sprayed with cooking spray.
- Bake eggplant for 15 minutes until tender.
- Layer eggplant slices with marinara, mozzarella, and Parmesan in a baking dish.
- Bake for another 5 minutes until cheese is melted.
- Garnish with fresh basil if desired.
- Serve and enjoy!

CHICKEN SOUP

PREP	COOK	SERVING SIZE	POINTS
10 Mins	25 Mins	1 cup	3

INGREDIENTS

- 1 lb boneless, skinless chicken breasts, diced
- 1 onion, diced
- 2 carrots, sliced
- 2 celery stalks, sliced
- 2 cloves garlic, minced
- 6 cups low-sodium chicken broth
- 1 teaspoon dried thyme
- 1 teaspoon dried rosemary
- Salt and pepper to taste
- 1 cup chopped spinach or kale
- Cooking spray

DIRECTIONS

- Spray a large pot with cooking spray, then sauté diced onion, carrots, celery, and minced garlic for about 5 minutes.
- Add diced chicken breasts and cook until no longer pink, about 5-7 minutes.
- Pour in chicken broth, add dried thyme, rosemary, salt, and pepper. Stir.
- Bring to a boil, then simmer for 15-20 minutes until vegetables are tender and flavors meld.
- Stir in chopped spinach or kale and cook for an additional 2-3 minutes until wilted.
- Adjust seasoning if necessary.
- Serve hot.

AFRICAN PEANUT SOUP

PREP
10 Mins

COOK
25 Mins

SERVING
4

POINTS
4

INGREDIENTS

- 1 tablespoon olive oil
- 1 medium onion, chopped
- 2 cloves garlic, minced
- 1 teaspoon grated ginger
- 1 teaspoon ground cumin
- 1 teaspoon ground coriander
- 1/4 teaspoon cayenne pepper (adjust to taste)
- 1 medium sweet potato, peeled and diced
- 4 cups vegetable broth (low-sodium if possible)
- 1 (14-ounce) can diced tomatoes, with juices
- 1/2 cup natural peanut butter (unsweetened)
- Salt and pepper to taste
- Fresh cilantro for garnish (optional)
- Chopped peanuts for garnish (optional)

DIRECTIONS

- Heat olive oil in a large pot over medium heat. Add chopped onion and cook until translucent, about 5 minutes.
- Add minced garlic and grated ginger, cook for another minute until fragrant.
- Stir in ground cumin, ground coriander, and cayenne pepper. Cook for another minute.
- Add diced sweet potato, vegetable broth, and diced tomatoes with their juices. Bring to a simmer and cook until sweet potatoes are tender, about 15-20 minutes.
- Stir in natural peanut butter until well combined and simmer for another 5 minutes.
- Taste and adjust seasoning with salt and pepper.
- Serve hot, garnished with fresh cilantro and chopped peanuts if desired.

CHILI-ROASTED CHICKEN AND POTATOES

PREP	**COOK**	**SERVING SIZE**	**POINTS**
10 Mins	30 Mins	1	5

INGREDIENTS

- 4 boneless, skinless chicken breasts
- 4 medium potatoes, washed and cubed
- 1 tablespoon olive oil
- 1 teaspoon chili powder
- 1/2 teaspoon garlic powder
- 1/2 teaspoon onion powder
- 1/2 teaspoon paprika
- Salt and pepper to taste

DIRECTIONS

- Preheat your oven to 400°F (200°C).
- Place chicken breasts and cubed potatoes in a large bowl. Drizzle with olive oil and sprinkle with chili powder, garlic powder, onion powder, paprika, salt, and pepper. Toss until chicken and potatoes are evenly coated with the seasoning mixture.
- Arrange the seasoned chicken breasts and potatoes in a single layer in a baking dish or on a baking sheet lined with parchment paper.
- Place the baking dish in the preheated oven and roast for about 25-30 minutes, or until the chicken is cooked through and the potatoes are tender, stirring halfway through.
- Let rest briefly, then serve hot.

SUMMER BERRY CREPE

PREP 10 Mins	**COOK** 20 Mins	**SERVING SIZE** 2	**POINTS** 7

INGREDIENTS

For the Crepes:

- 1/2 cup all-purpose flour
- 1 large egg
- 1/2 cup unsweetened almond milk (or any milk of your choice)
- 1 tablespoon unsalted butter, melted
- 1/2 teaspoon vanilla extract
- Cooking spray or additional butter for the pan

For the Filling:

- 1/2 cup mixed berries (such as strawberries, blueberries, raspberries)
- 1 teaspoon lemon juice
- 1 teaspoon honey or maple syrup (optional)
- Greek yogurt or low-fat whipped cream for serving (optional)

DIRECTIONS

- In a mixing bowl, whisk together the flour, egg, almond milk, melted butter, and vanilla extract until smooth and well combined. Let the batter rest for about 10 minutes.
- Heat a non-stick skillet or crepe pan over medium heat. Lightly coat the skillet with cooking spray or melt a small amount of butter.
- Pour about 1/4 cup of the crepe batter into the skillet, swirling it around to coat the bottom evenly. Cook for about 1-2 minutes, or until the edges start to lift and the bottom is lightly golden.
- Carefully flip the crepe using a spatula and cook for an additional 1-2 minutes on the other side. Repeat with the remaining batter,

- stacking the cooked crepes on a plate and covering them with a clean kitchen towel to keep warm.
- In a small bowl, toss the mixed berries with lemon juice and honey or maple syrup (if using). Set aside.
- Place one crepe on a serving plate. Spoon some of the mixed berry filling onto one half of the crepe, then fold it in half to enclose the filling. Fold in half again to form a triangle shape.
- Repeat with the remaining crepes and berry filling.
- Serve the summer berry crepes with a dollop of Greek yogurt or low-fat whipped cream, if desired.

TOMATO AND RED ONION SALSA

PREP
10 Mins

COOK
0 Mins

SERVING SIZE
4

POINTS
0

INGREDIENTS

Tomato
- 3 Large, halved and seeded, flesh finely chopped

Red onion
- 1 medium, thinly sliced

Chili, green or red
- 1 individual, red, deseeded and chopped

Coriander, fresh
- 2 tablespoon(s), finely chopped, plus extra to serve

Lime Juice, Fresh
- 1 tablespoon(s)

DIRECTIONS

- Halve and deseed 3 large tomatoes, then finely chop the flesh. Combine the tomatoes with 1 thinly sliced red onion, 1 deseeded and chopped red chilli, 2 tablespoons finely chopped fresh coriander and the juice of ½ lime in a small bowl, then season to taste and serve with extra finely chopped fresh coriander sprinkled over the top.

TURKEY BURGERS

PREP 10 Mins	**COOK** 10 Mins	**SERVING SIZE** 4	**POINTS** 0

INGREDIENTS

- 1 lb fat-free ground turkey (97%-99% lean)
- ½ cup salsa
- 1½ teaspoon chili powder
- Salt & pepper to taste
- ½ cup panko crumbs
- 2 oz (½ cup) reduced-fat shredded mozzarella

DIRECTIONS

- In a bowl mix your ground turkey, panko, salsa, chili powder, salt and pepper together.

- Portion into 4 burgers then roll each section into a ball. Push a hole into the middle of the ball, add the cheese, then roll back into a ball. Pat the burger down until flat and in a burger shape.

- Cook on a grill until internal temp reaches 165 degrees. You can also cook in a skillet on the stove or in an oven at 400 degrees.

Exercises that aid Weight loss

JUMPING JACKS

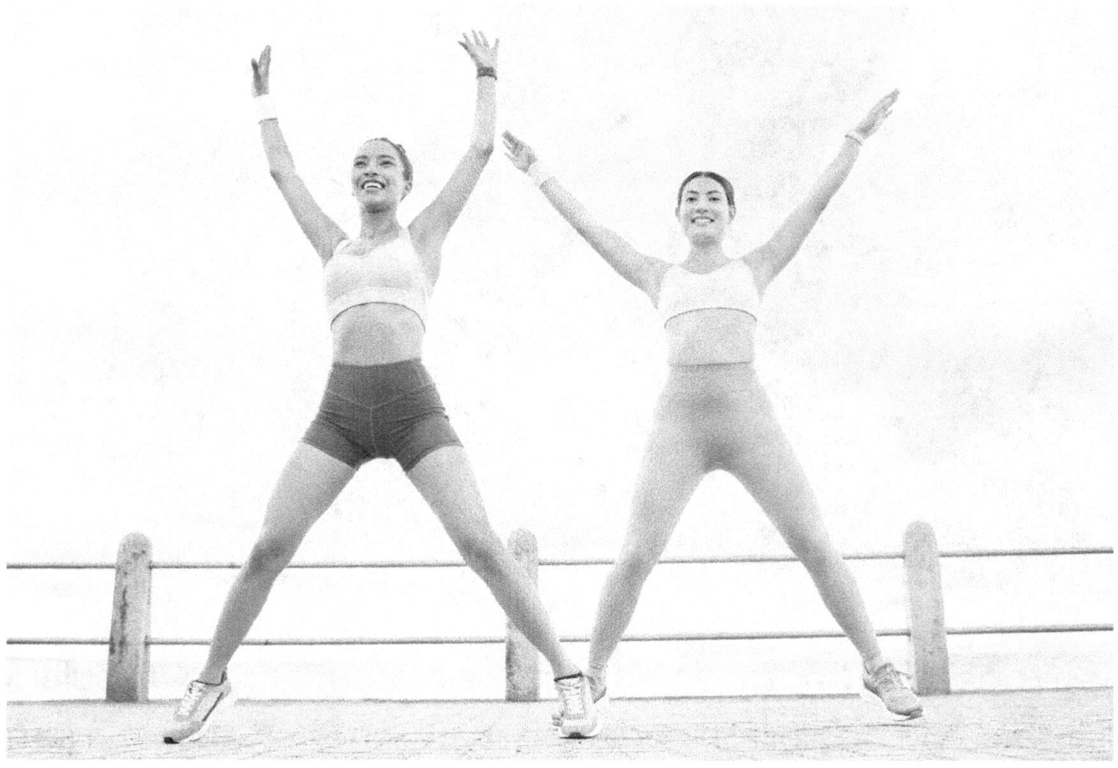

Jumping jacks are a simple and effective cardiovascular exercise.
Here's how to perform them:

1. Start Position: Stand with your feet together and your arms at your sides.
2. Jump Out: Jump your feet out to the sides while simultaneously raising your arms above your head. Your hands should meet above your head at the top of the jump, or you can clap your hands together.
3. Return to Start: Jump back to the starting position by bringing your feet together and lowering your arms back to your sides.
4. Repeat: Continue jumping in and out, keeping a steady rhythm.

JUMP ROPE

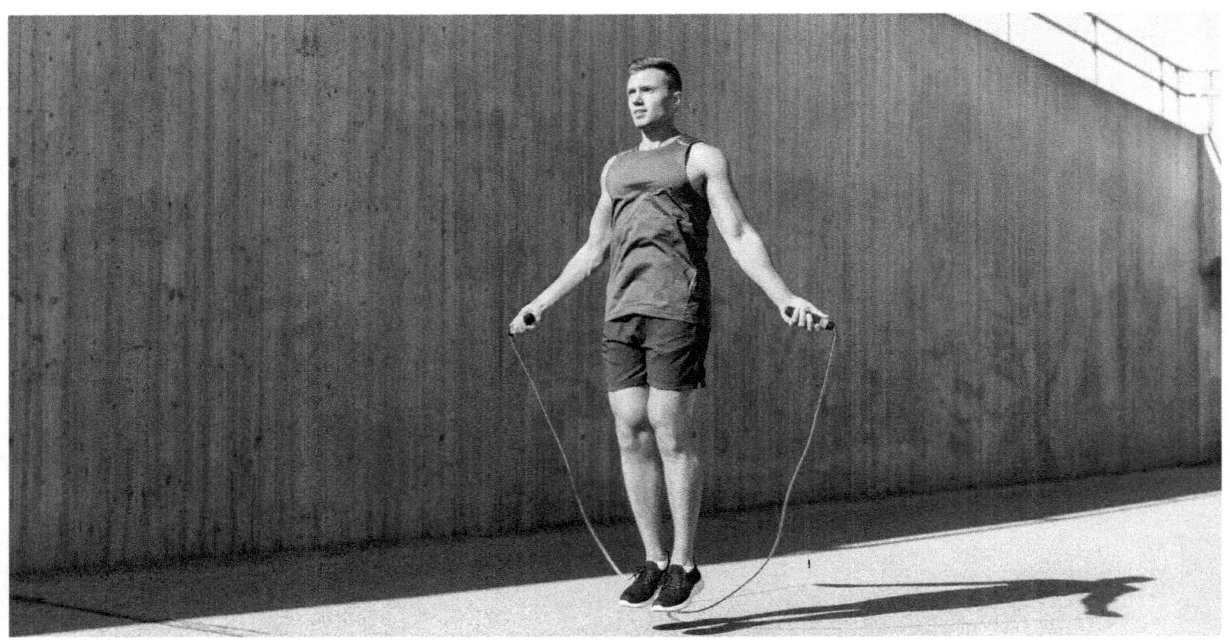

Jumping rope, also known as skipping, is a great cardiovascular exercise that can be performed almost anywhere with just a jump rope. Here's a basic guide on how to perform jump rope:

- Get the Right Rope: Choose a rope that suits your height.
- Find Space: Clear a flat area to jump.
- Proper Form: Hold the handles, keep knees slightly bent, and jump with both feet.
- Start Basic: Practice basic jumps first.
- Timing: Jump to the rhythm of the rope.
- Variations: Try different jumps once you're comfortable.
- Safety: Land softly, avoid hard surfaces, and listen to your body.
- Cool Down: Stretch after your workout.
- Consistency: Practice regularly to improve.

MOUNTAIN CLIMBERS

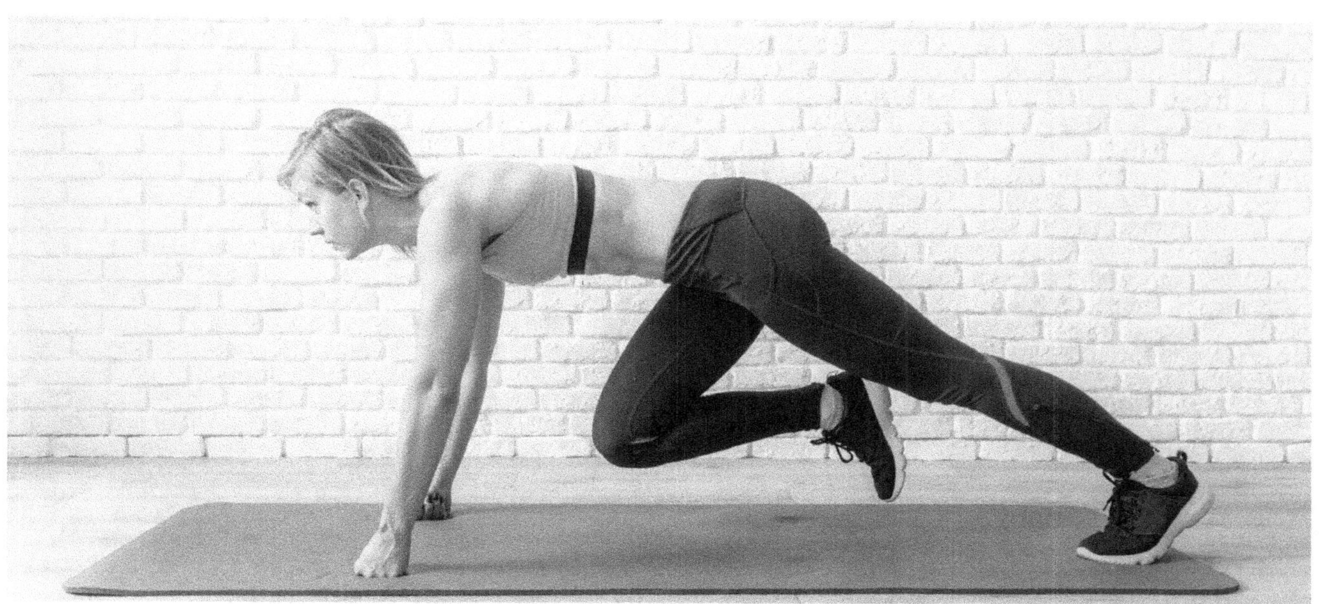

1. Starting Position: Begin in a high plank position with hands flat on the ground shoulder-width apart and body forming a straight line from head to heels.
2. Drive Knee Towards Chest: Lift your right foot off the ground and drive your right knee towards your chest, engaging your core.
3. Switch Legs: Quickly switch legs, jumping or hopping so your left knee is now driving towards your chest while your right leg extends back.
4. Repeat: Alternate legs in a smooth, controlled manner, maintaining a steady rhythm.
5. Breathing: Inhale and exhale steadily as you perform the movement, exhaling as you drive your knee towards your chest.
6. Complete Reps or Time: Perform for a certain number of repetitions or duration, starting with manageable numbers and increasing gradually.

SQUAT JUMPS

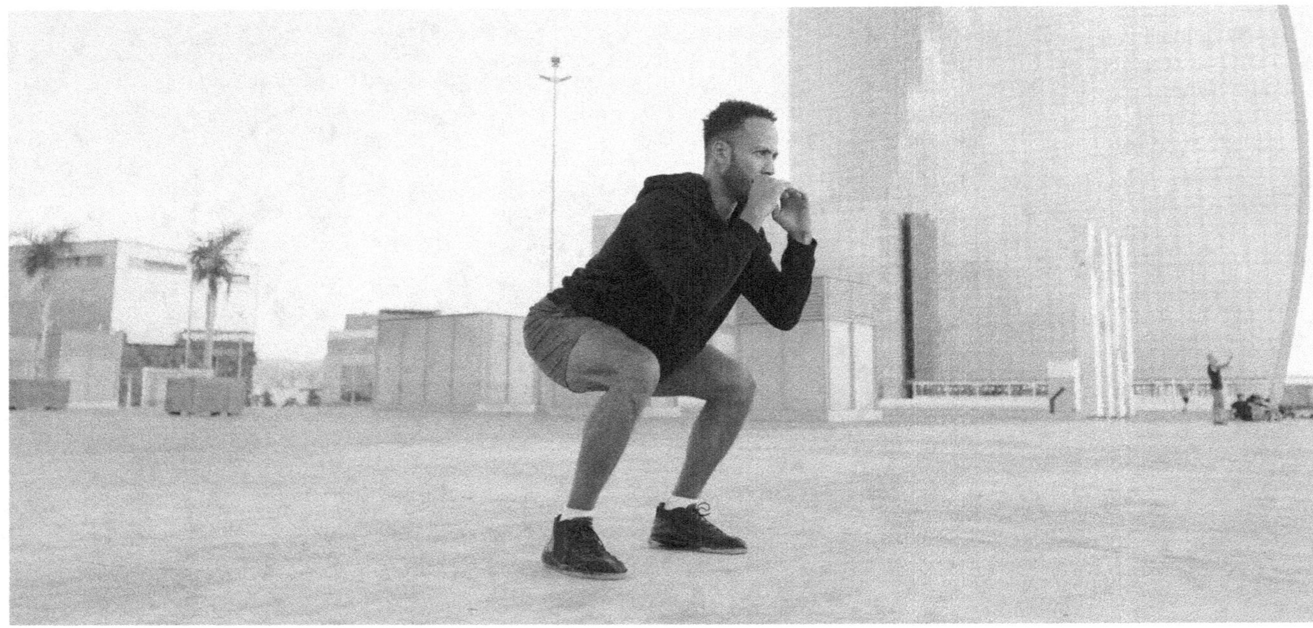

1. Stand with your feet shoulder-width apart, toes pointing slightly outward.
2. Lower your body into a squat position by bending your knees and pushing your hips back.
3. Keep your chest up and your back straight.
4. Explosively jump upward as high as you can from the squat position.
5. As you jump, extend your arms overhead for balance and momentum.
6. Land softly back into the squat position, absorbing the impact with your knees bent.
7. Repeat the movement for the desired number of repetitions or time.

LUNGES

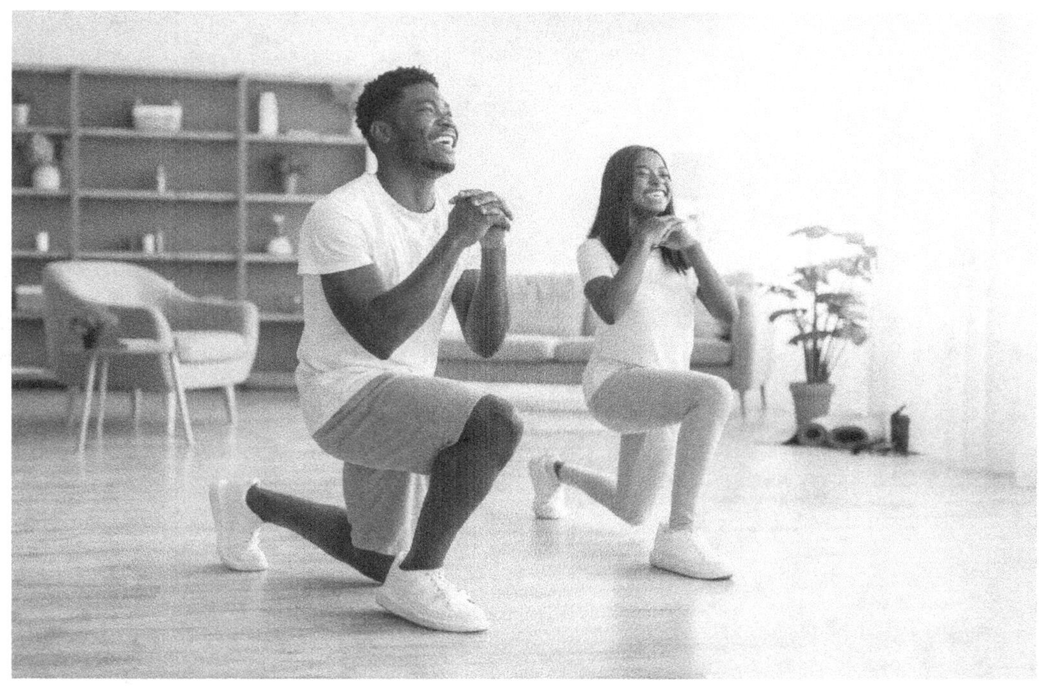

To perform lunges:

1. Stand up straight with your feet hip-width apart.
2. Take a step forward with one leg, lowering your hips until both knees are bent at about a 90-degree angle.
3. Keep your front knee directly above your ankle, and your back knee just above the floor without touching it.
4. Push back up to the starting position using your front heel.
5. Repeat with the opposite leg.

Remember to keep your torso upright and engage your core muscles throughout the exercise.`

SIDE PLANK

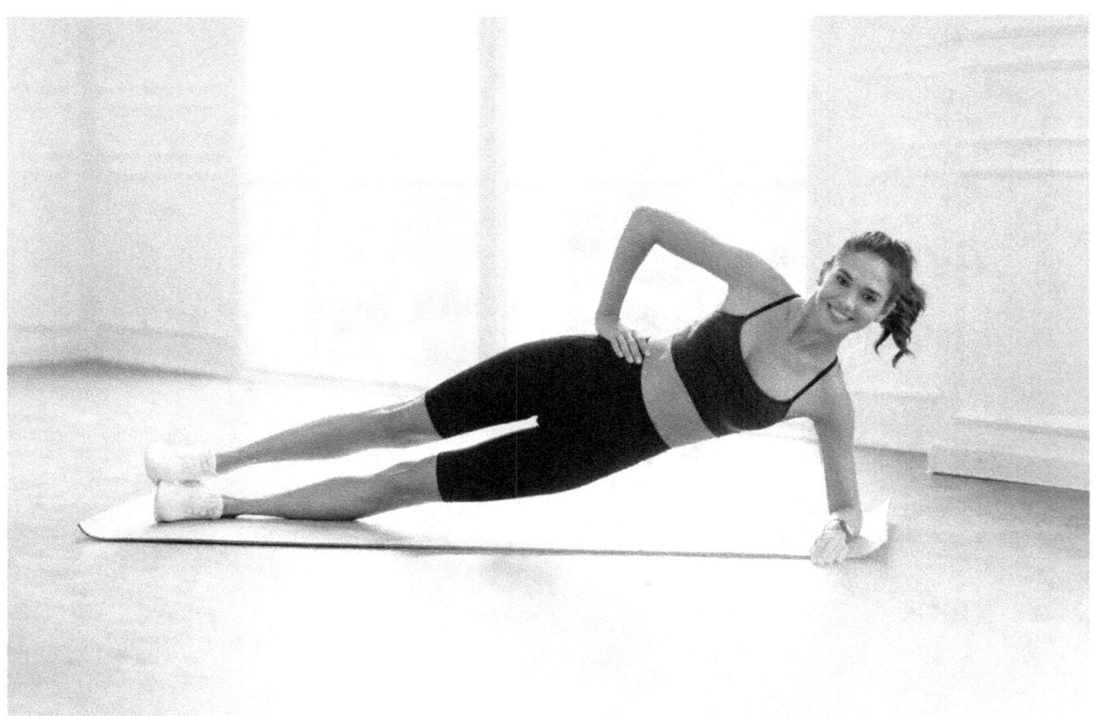

To perform a Side Plank:

1. Start by lying on your side with your legs extended.
2. Prop yourself up on your forearm, keeping your elbow directly beneath your shoulder.
3. Lift your hips off the ground, creating a straight line from your head to your feet.
4. Engage your core muscles to maintain stability.
5. Hold this position for the desired amount of time, typically aiming for 20-60 seconds.
6. Switch sides and repeat.

REVERSE PLANK

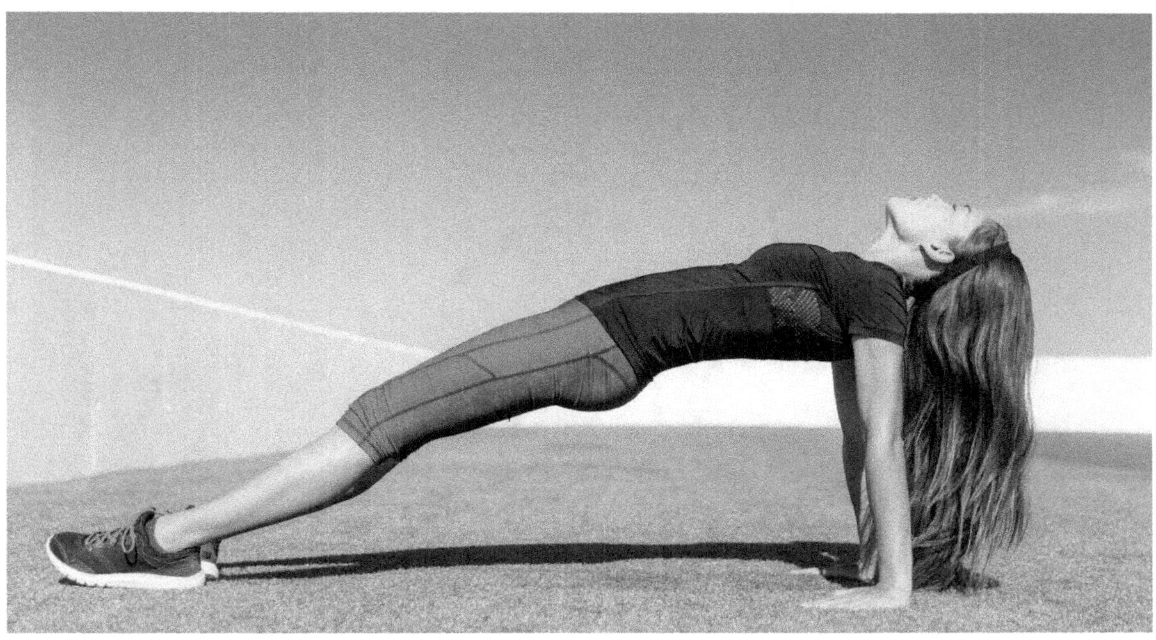

To perform a Reverse Plank:

1. Sit on the floor with your legs extended in front of you.
2. Place your hands on the floor slightly behind your hips, fingers pointing toward your feet.
3. Press into your palms and lift your hips toward the ceiling, creating a straight line from your head to your heels.
4. Keep your chest open and shoulders down, engaging your core and glutes.
5. Hold the position for the desired duration, then lower your hips back to the floor to release.

Remember to breathe steadily throughout the exercise and avoid overarching your lower back.

PUSH-UPS

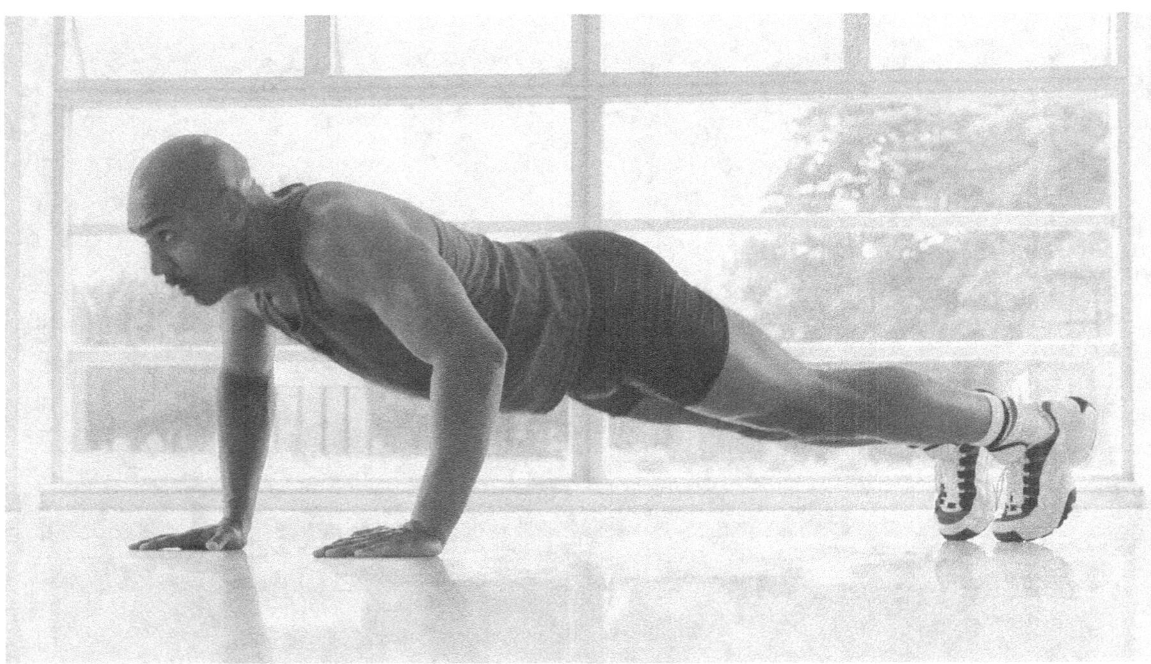

Here's a quick guide on how to perform push-ups:

1. Start in a plank position, with your hands slightly wider than shoulder-width apart and your arms fully extended.
2. Keep your body in a straight line from head to heels, engaging your core and glutes.
3. Lower your body by bending your elbows until your chest nearly touches the ground.
4. Keep your elbows close to your body, not flared out to the sides.
5. Push through your palms to straighten your arms, returning to the starting position.
6. Repeat for the desired number of repetitions.

BICYCLE CRUNCHES

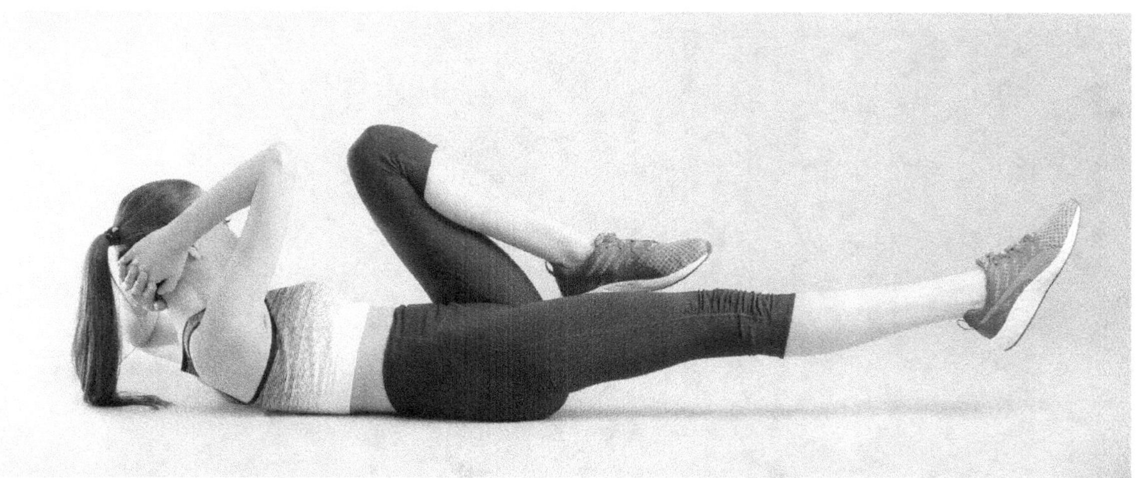

To perform Bicycle Crunches:

1. Lie on your back with your hands behind your head, elbows pointing outward.
2. Lift your legs off the ground, bending them at the knees to form a 90-degree angle.
3. Lift your shoulders off the ground, engaging your core.
4. Begin by straightening your left leg out while simultaneously twisting your torso to bring your right elbow towards your left knee.
5. Alternate sides by bending your right leg and straightening your left leg while twisting your torso to bring your left elbow towards your right knee.
6. Continue alternating sides in a pedaling motion while keeping your core engaged throughout the exercise.
7. Aim for controlled movements and avoid pulling on your neck with your hands.
8. Repeat for the desired number of repetitions.

HIGH KNEES

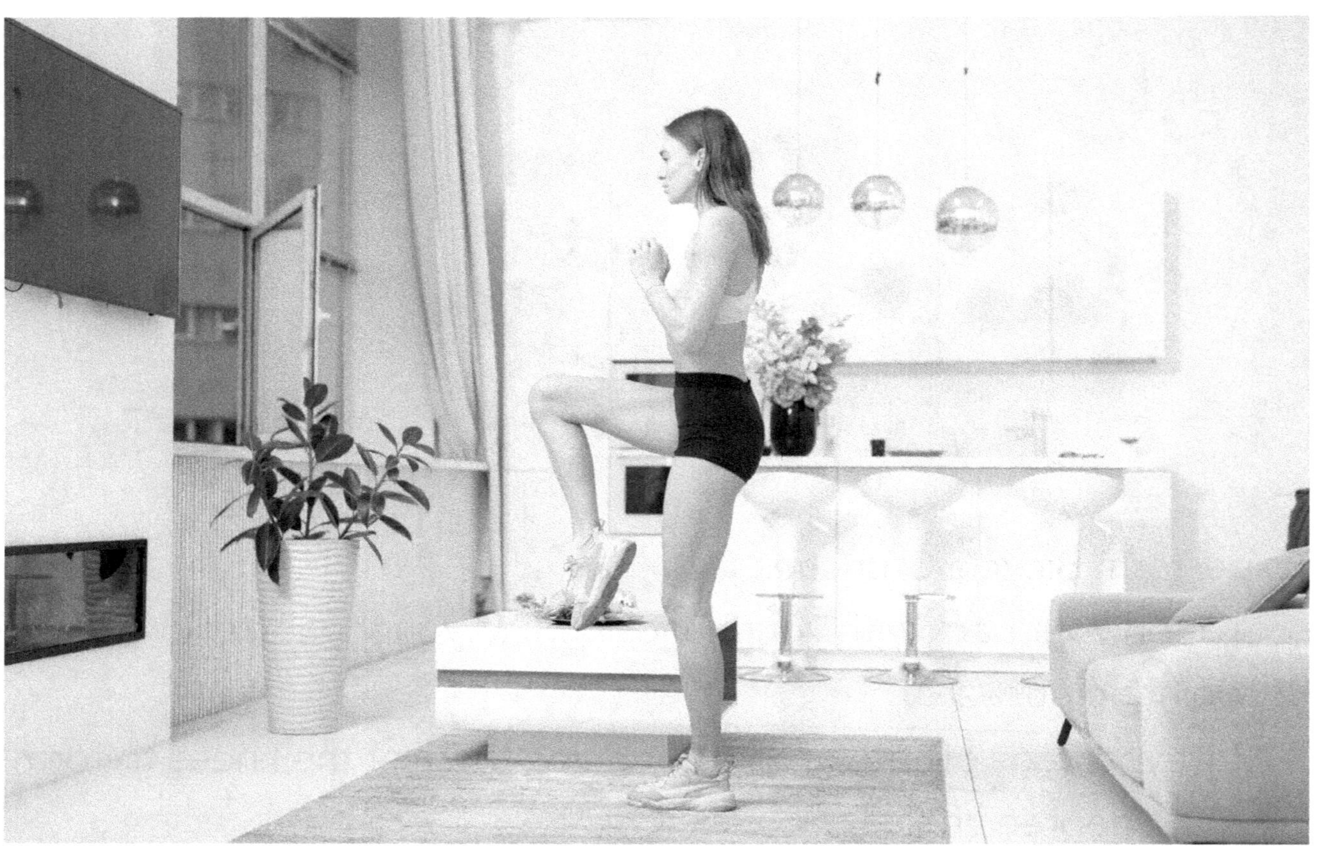

To perform High Knees:

1. Stand upright with your feet hip-width apart.
2. Lift your right knee up towards your chest as high as possible, while simultaneously driving your left arm forward.
3. Quickly switch, lowering your right leg and lifting your left knee towards your chest, while driving your right arm forward.
4. Continue alternating legs at a fast pace, as if you are jogging in place, bringing your knees up as high as you can with each step.

WALKING

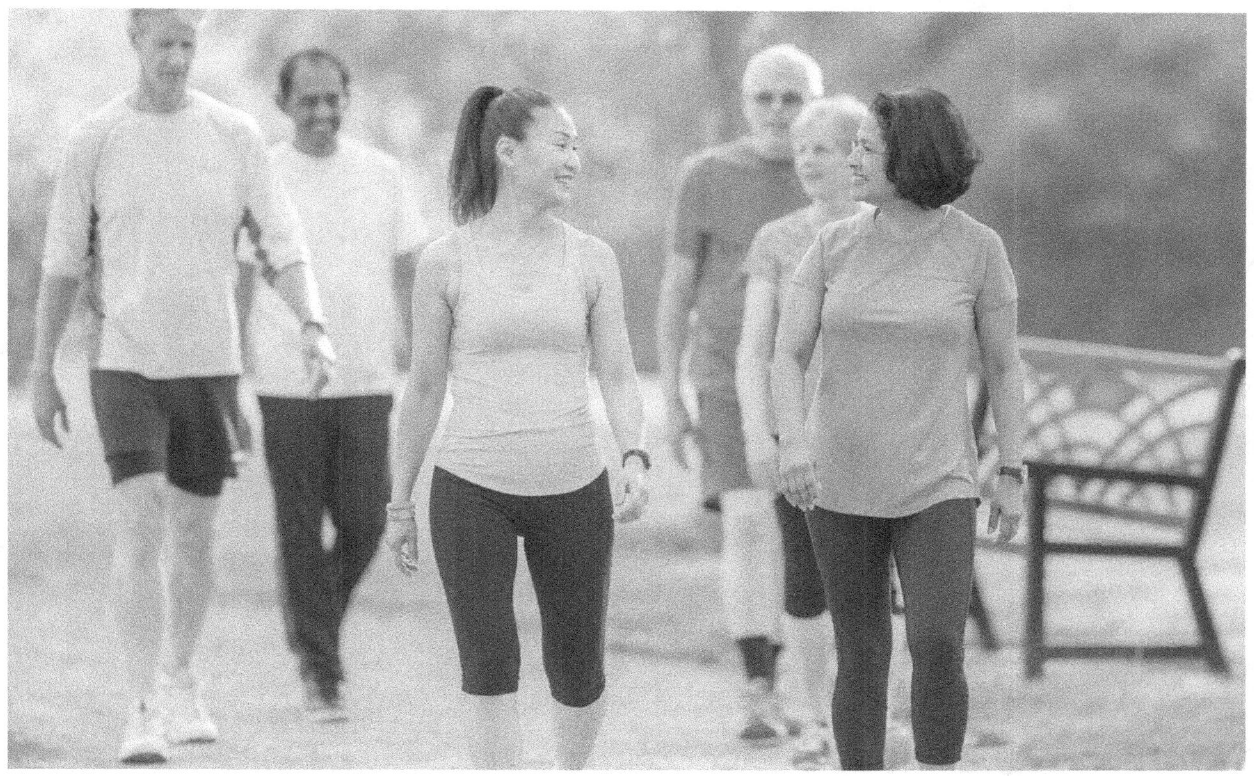

To perform walking:

1. Stand upright with your feet shoulder-width apart.
2. Keep your head up and look forward.
3. Swing your arms naturally at your sides.
4. Take a step forward with your right foot, followed by your left foot.
5. Continue alternating steps, maintaining a steady pace.
6. Land on your heel and roll through the step to push off with your toes.
7. Keep your core engaged for balance.
8. Maintain a relaxed posture and breathe steadily.
9. Walk in a straight line, avoiding excessive swaying or leaning.
10. Enjoy your walk and stay aware of your surroundings for safety.

WALL SITS

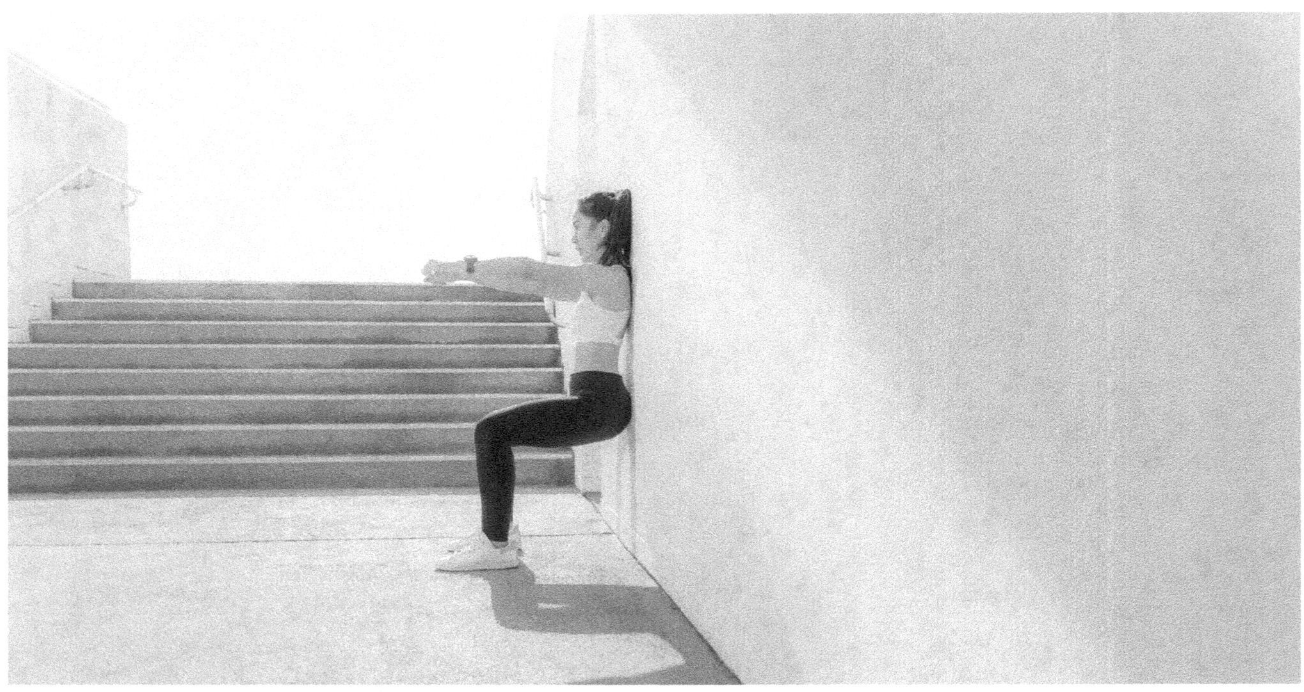

Performing a wall sit is relatively simple:

1. Find a clear wall space.
2. Stand with your back against the wall.
3. Lower your body until your thighs are parallel to the ground, as if you were sitting on an invisible chair.
4. Keep your back flat against the wall and your knees at a 90-degree angle.
5. Hold this position for as long as you can, aiming for at least 30 seconds to start.
6. Focus on keeping your core engaged and your weight in your heels.
7. When you're ready to finish, stand up slowly.

BOX JUMPS

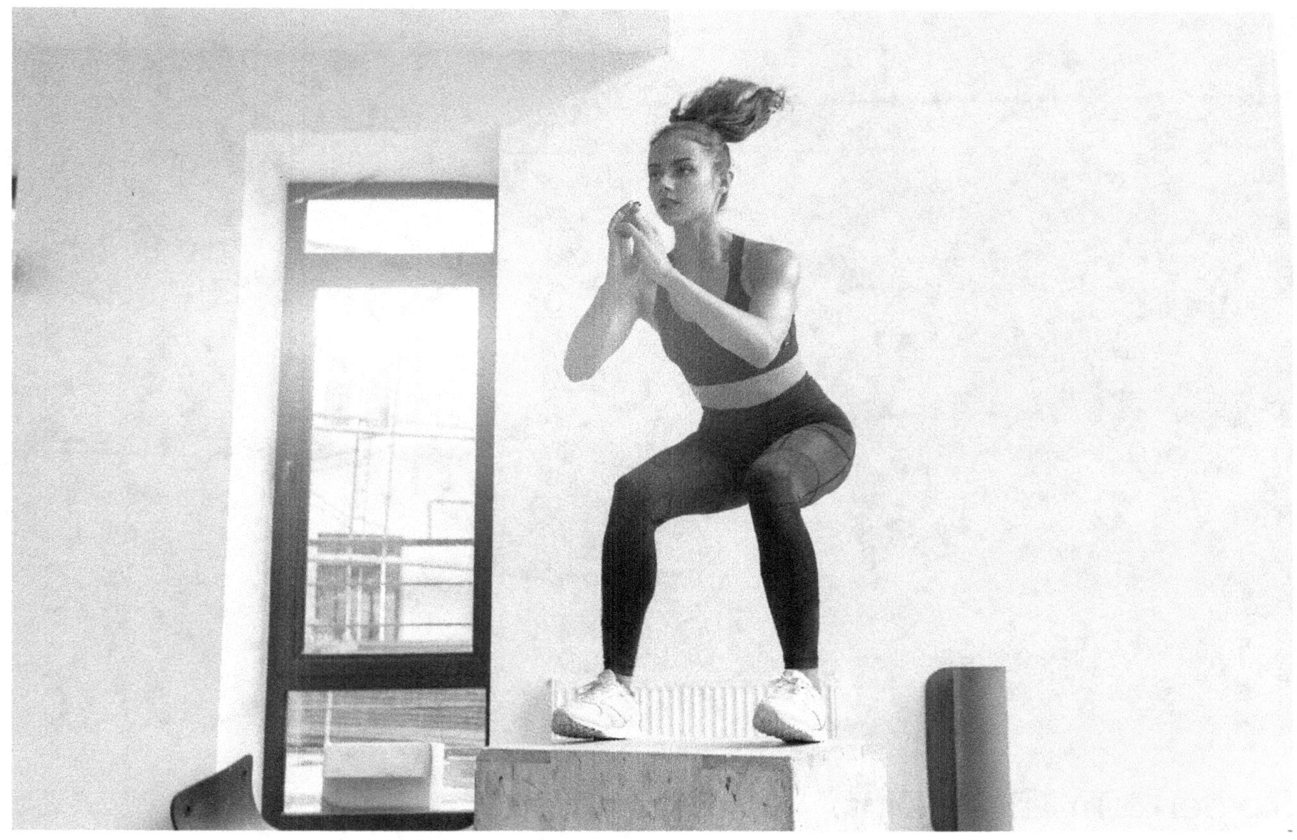

To perform box jumps:

1. Stand facing a sturdy box or platform of a height suitable for your fitness level.
2. Start with your feet shoulder-width apart.
3. Bend your knees and swing your arms back.
4. Explosively jump onto the box, swinging your arms forward for momentum.
5. Land softly on the box, using your hips and knees to absorb the impact.
6. Stand tall on top of the box for a moment.
7. Step or jump down carefully, landing softly with bent knees.
8. Repeat for the desired number of repetitions.

TRICEP DIPS

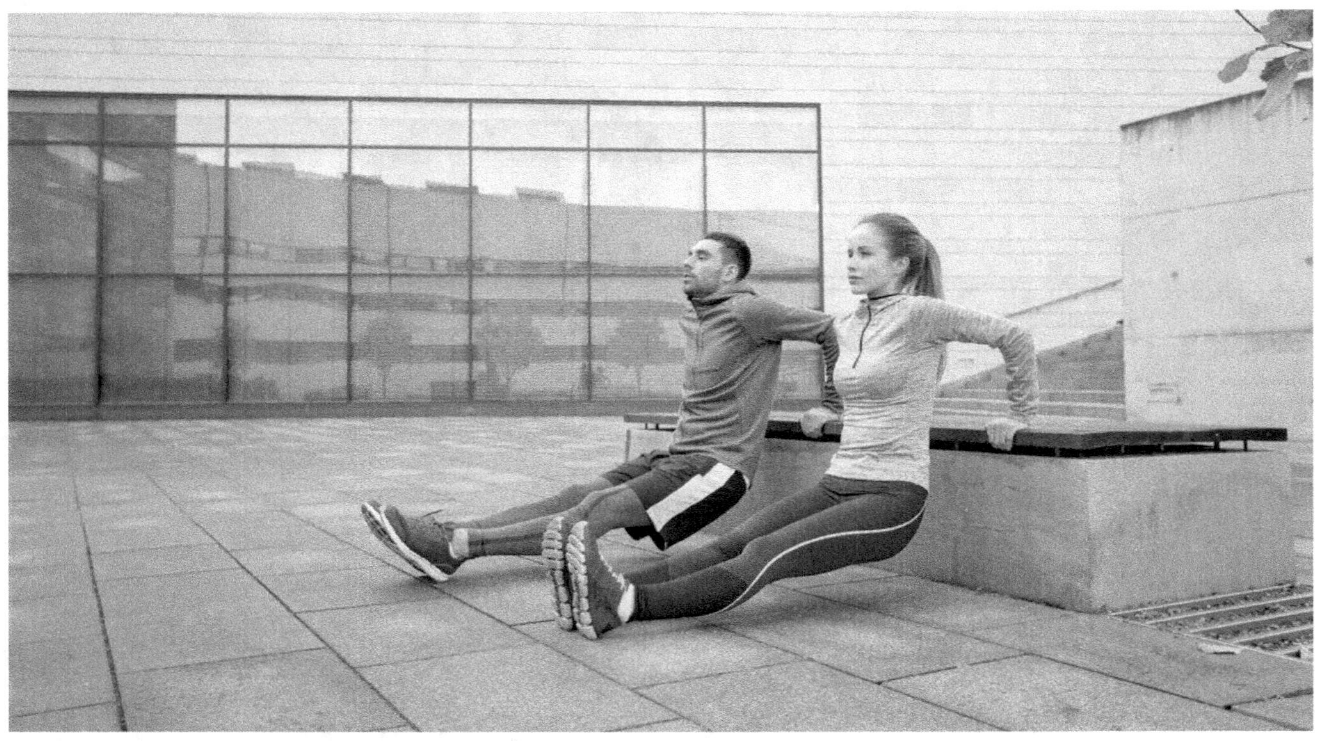

To perform Tricep Dips:

1. Sit on the edge of a sturdy chair or bench.
2. Place your hands shoulder-width apart on the edge of the chair or bench, fingers gripping the edge.
3. Slide your butt off the front of the chair or bench, supporting your weight with your hands.
4. Keep your legs extended in front of you or bent at the knees for a modified version.
5. Lower your body by bending your elbows until your upper arms are parallel to the ground.
6. Push yourself back up to the starting position by straightening your arms, but don't lock your elbows.
7. Repeat for the desired number of reps.

BEAR CRAWLS

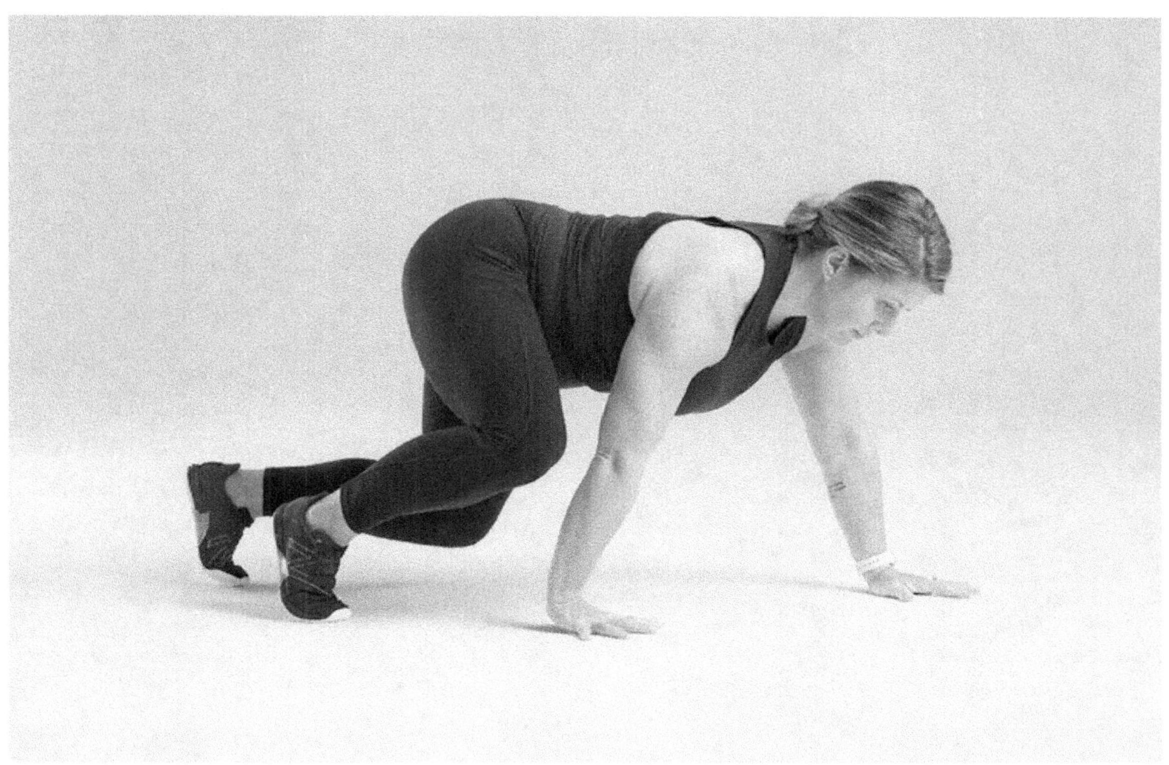

To perform Bear Crawls:

1. Start in a tabletop position with your hands directly under your shoulders and your knees under your hips.
2. Lift your knees a few inches off the ground, keeping your back flat and core engaged.
3. Move forward by stepping your right hand and left foot simultaneously, followed by your left hand and right foot.
4. Keep your movements controlled and steady, maintaining a stable core throughout.
5. Continue crawling forward for a set distance or time, then reverse the movement to crawl backward if desired.

BURPEES

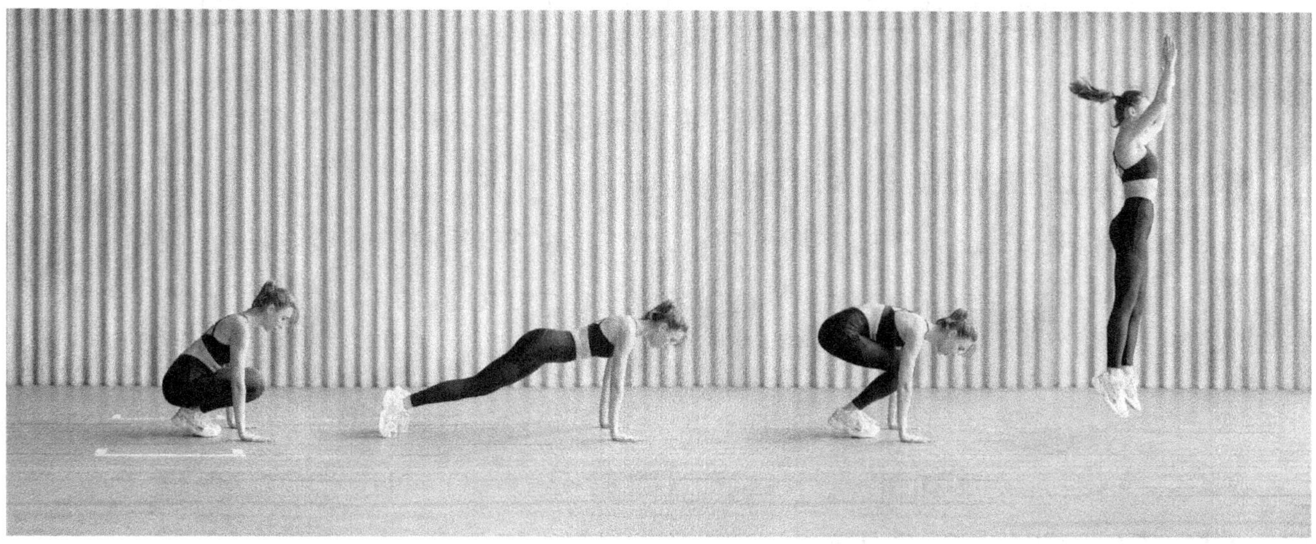

Burpees are a high-intensity, full-body exercise that combines elements of strength training and aerobic conditioning. Here's a step-by-step guide on how to perform a basic burpee:

- Start Position: Stand with your feet shoulder-width apart, arms at your sides.
- Squat: Lower your body into a squat position by bending your knees and pushing your hips back, keeping your back straight and chest up.
- Kick Back: From the squat position, kick your feet back into a plank position, keeping your arms extended and hands shoulder-width apart. Your body should be in a straight line from head to heels, engaging your core muscles to maintain stability.
- Push-Up: Perform one push-up, lowering your chest towards the ground by bending your elbows while keeping your body in a straight line. You can modify this by dropping to your knees if needed.

- Return to Squat Position: After completing the push-up, jump your feet back towards your hands, returning to the squat position.
- Jump Up: Explode upwards into a jump, reaching your arms overhead as you leave the ground.
- Land Softly: Land softly on your feet and immediately lower back into the squat position to begin the next repetition.

Here are some tips to keep in mind while performing burpees:

1. Focus on maintaining proper form throughout the exercise to prevent injury and maximize effectiveness.
2. Engage your core muscles to stabilize your body during each phase of the burpee.
3. Keep a steady pace to maintain intensity throughout your workout.
4. Modify the exercise as needed based on your fitness level. You can start with a modified version by skipping the push-up or the jump if necessary.
5. Incorporate burpees into your workout routine as part of a circuit or interval training for a challenging full-body workout.